21 POUNDS *in* 21 DAYS

21 POUNDS in 21 DAYS

The Martha's Vineyard Diet Detox

RONI DeLUZ, RN, ND, PhD

With **JAMES HESTER** and **HILARY BEARD**

HARPER

NEW YORK • LONDON • TORONTO • SYDNEY

To my dear children, Whitney, Toron, and Tony, Jr.: I pray that you learn early in life that God's love is like no other, and that cleansing your body and mind clears the pathway for the best things in life to come to you.

To all of my clients: You are all very special and have become dear to me. I truly enjoy my life and it's because of you.

Roni DeLuz is a registered nurse, traditional naturopathic doctor, PhD in natural healing, lifestyle consultant, certified colon therapist, and hypnotherapist. She is not a medical physician, psychologist or pharmacist, and as such, this book is a source of information only, and not a substitute for the advice of the reader's personal physician or other medical professional, who should be consulted before beginning any diet regimen and before taking any herbs or supplements.

All efforts have been made to ensure the accuracy of the information contained in this book as of the date published. The author and the publisher expressly disclaim responsibility for any adverse effects arising from the use or application of the information contained in this book.

HarperCollins books may be purchased for educational, business, or sales promotional use. For information please write: Special Markets Department, HarperCollins Publishers, 10 East 53rd Street, New York, NY 10022.

First Collins paperback edition published 2008

Designed by Nancy Peng Singer

Library of Congress Cataloging-in-Publication Data is available upon request.

ISBN 978-0-06-124209-0 (pbk.)

10 11 12 13 14   ID/RRD   10 9 8 7 6

CONTENTS

PREFACE BY ALBERTO MARTINEZ, MD   vii

INTRODUCTION   1

     Testimonial James Hester   16

1   Toxic, Unhealthy, and Heavy: America's Rude Awakening   23

2   Detoxing vs. Dieting: What's the Difference?   53

     Testimonial Marcia Buckley   78

3   The Martha's Vineyard Diet Detox: Reduce, Rejuvenate, and Rebuild   81

     Testimonial The Three Sisters   97

4   All About Juices and Soups   101

5   Supplements You'll Need During the Detox   117

     Testimonial Rosalie Forest   124

6   Understanding Elimination Therapy   127

7   Setting Up for Success   153

     Testimonial Judi Thompson   168

8   Doing the Detox   173

     Testimonial Hilary Beard   185

9   Ending the Detox   191

RECIPES   205

GLOSSARY   213

ACKNOWLEDGMENTS   217

INDEX   225

PREFACE

In 2004 I met Dr. Roni DeLuz by phone when she called to discuss my approach to treating infectious diseases and other chronic and degenerative problems. Dr. Roni had heard about me from some of her patients, at least one of whom I had treated in my clinic in Juarez, Mexico (I also have an office in El Paso, Texas). While I am a traditional medical doctor—I am trained as a general practitioner, though I completed postgraduate studies at Columbia University in New York in parasitology and public health—I have worked in several parts of the world, where I have been exposed to healing treatments that are either unavailable or not widely practiced in the United States. Throughout Europe, medical professionals employ a wide range of approaches that can be considered complementary therapies. I have lived and practiced in England, which I consider to be the prototype of a modern society where alternative therapies are taking hold. The British medical system has implemented a permanent program to provide its citizens with information on alternative therapies, such as acupuncture, homeopathy, osteopathy, and herbal medicine, in every public medical setting. In Germany, many practitioners perform in what Americans consider alternative fields. In England, as well as in Belgium, the Netherlands, and other countries, I have set up clinics and trained doctors how to perform chelation and ozone therapies, treatments not practiced by American medical doctors. As a result of this type of exposure and additional training I have received, I take a different approach from the orthodox way many American medical doctors treat patients. Dr. Roni knew this.

Over two or three months Dr. Roni and I spoke several times, during which we spoke about the kind of work we do in our respective practices. Eventually, she asked if she could come to visit me in Mexico so she could see what I do. I happily said yes. After meeting her and learning that she had some medical problems, I offered to treat her. In exchange, she offered the same. My goal was to lose 8 to 10 pounds. I had been a long-distance runner for many years—I've run in the New York City marathon three times. But between working long hours and being single, I had begun to become less disciplined about eating and had gained a little weight.

So when I went to Dr. Roni's retreat in Massachusetts in January 2004, I already knew quite a bit about her work. But I was quite surprised to discover how deep and comprehensive her protocol—her approach—is. I detoxed for 16 straight days, which was as long as I could afford to stay away from my practice. To be honest, in the beginning I found detoxing difficult. During the first 5 or 6 days, I was about to quit and say goodbye. I didn't like the eating restrictions, I felt isolated from my work and patients, and I have to admit I was uncomfortable with the roles being reversed—I was used to being the caretaker, not the person being taken care of. But after 6 or 7 days, my state of mind began to ease. I began to feel reconciled with the approach. Then it got kind of fun. It was really rewarding to see the changes. I was losing a pound per day. I was feeling better physically—I was actually feeling very good. My spirits were better and I felt more optimistic. A mental well-being that apparently I had lost suddenly returned to me. By the end of the 16 days, I had shed 16 pounds. It was absolutely amazing!

As both a medical doctor and someone who has experienced the Martha's Vineyard Diet Detox firsthand, I know that Dr. Roni's approach is a good one. It looks at the person holistically rather than focusing on just their health problem. It helps people confront themselves, their habits, and the behaviors that have caused the problem. And it helps them to lose weight, prevent disease, or regain health, depending on their circumstances. I particularly recommend it for people who have problems with overeating and obesity. The program offers what could be a once-in-a-lifetime opportunity for people to experience a fresh start, a new beginning that can help prevent health problems or the recurrence of existing ones, and to learn how to nourish themselves properly for life. This is particularly true for those who are able to go to Dr. Roni's clinic.

I believe that anyone who needs to regain health *should* do the Martha's Vineyard Diet Detox. Many times, we can improve our health naturally. That is the key part—naturally. I think it's important to accomplish what we can by using the most naturally oriented approaches to preventing or eliminating excess weight and diseases. Rather than relying on "quick fixes," medication, or medical interventions to help us get or stay healthy, I believe in practicing prevention and supporting our body's own ability to heal itself. By educating ourselves about proper nutrition and by learning how important it is to have the proper intake of the right foods, we empower ourselves to improve our health for the rest of our lives.

I believe that Dr. Roni's approach is the right approach for dealing with excess weight and related problems. Though we medical professionals are often wary about complementary and alternative approaches, I think we must also exhibit openness. Particularly in the United States, I believe there is a lot of work to be done in that regard. Fortunately, I believe this is starting to happen; I have seen many American doctors and practitioners overseas, learning what is happening in other countries. We should not close our eyes to alternative approaches that work. The Martha's Vineyard Diet Detox works. I highly recommend it.

Alberto Martinez, MD
El Paso, Texas

INTRODUCTION

The Martha's Vineyard Diet Detox is not a traditional weight-loss program. You will definitely lose weight, but unlike when you diet, you won't feel hungry, experience cravings, or later experience the yo-yo effect of dropping 10 pounds and then gaining back 15. You won't have to count calories, points, indices, or rankings, or do anything else that requires math. There are no bland or repetitive foods, like grapefruit, grapefruit, grapefruit. You won't spend a lot of money. And I promise not to make you squeeze into any Spandex.

The Martha's Vineyard Diet Detox is a *cleansing detoxification program*. We're all familiar with people detoxing from drugs and alcohol, but we rarely think of cleansing our bodies of other noxious substances. Yet we're all exposed to them daily in the environment and our homes and workplaces. Substances like cigarette smoke; smokestack emissions; pesticide runoff; carpet, paint, and bleach fumes; artificial flavors, colors, and preservatives; antibiotics and hormones; dry-cleaning fluid residue; nail polish; and hair color harm our body and compromise our well-being. Over time, toxic elements accumulate in our cells, gunk up our organs, erode our quality of life, and cause many of the low-grade discomforts that are all too familiar to many of us—allergies, fatigue, heartburn, headaches, and a loss of energy. Toxins make us more susceptible to serious chronic diseases like high blood pressure and diabetes. In fact, these poisons foul up the delicate inner workings of many people's bodies so much that they gain unwanted weight and it becomes nearly impossible for them to slim down. Many overweight people know from experience that weight loss is often about a lot more than eating the right foods and counting calories. For many, toxins are interfering with their bodily functions so much that being fat is not their fault!

In this book you will learn how to detoxify your body, purposefully flushing many poisonous substances out of your system. As you detoxify, you will naturally lose weight—no starving, no counting, no Spandex! The average person who does the Martha's Vineyard Diet Detox for 21 days loses 21 pounds. They do so safely, healthily, and with no yo-yo effect. Depending on how fast their metabolism is, many people lose even more weight. Some (mostly men; I'll explain why later) lose upwards of 30 pounds. People who detox for shorter time frames lose less. As they eliminate toxins, many people relieve or even heal themselves of annoying and even chronic health conditions that have been undermining their quality of life.

In these pages you will find three detoxifying weight-loss programs to pick from: the 21-day Diet Detox, the 7-day Tune-Up, and 2-day Weekend Cleanse. While I recommend that everyone follow the 21-day Diet Detox at least once yearly and/or the 7-day Tune-Up seasonally and/or the 2-day Weekend Cleanse, you can pick the program that feels most comfortable and achievable given your goals, lifestyle, and commitment level. Serious about shedding 20 pounds and improving your eating habits once and for all? Want to jump-start major weight loss? Need to lose weight because your health is at stake? Try the 21-day detox. Want to lose the 10 pounds that crept onto your waistline over the winter? The 7-day plan will get you close quickly. Feeling a little out of sorts because you lived it up on your birthday? Give the 2-day clean-up a whirl. Even if you decide to adopt just a few of the healthy habits I describe, you'll shed toxins for sure, and a few pounds along with them. You'll also experience clearer thinking; shed anger, guilt, and stress; and alleviate allergies and any propensity you have to retain fluids. And here's some good news: the Martha's Vineyard Diet Detox is not "all or nothing"—you don't have to do it perfectly. We'll show you how to "cheat" and get back on board. Even if you don't follow every step, you'll still lose weight, release toxins, and improve your well-being (although at a slower pace).

No matter which detox you select, you'll look and feel younger. Since the Martha's Vineyard Diet Detox stimulates your body to produce fresh new cells at a remarkably rapid rate, it is more antiaging than any expensive wrinkle cream you can buy at a department store or any scrub or peel from a chi-chi spa. It will literally turn back the clock on your body and your life. If you're like most people, you believe that wrinkles, memory loss, fatigue, arthritis, and vision loss are natural and inevitable symptoms of growing older. Well, I've got news: they're usually sure signs of a body that is overburdened with toxins. The Martha's Vineyard Diet Detox will relieve these symptoms in a remarkably short period of time. You will feel more energetic within 1 to 2 days. Your skin will become supple within a week, and acne will start to clear up. Your eyes will become brighter and begin to sparkle. Any yellowness in the whites of your eyes or excess "baggage" or "raccoon circles" under them will diminish within days. As you progress through the 21 days, your fingernails will strengthen and lengthen; your hair will grow quicker, longer, and shinier; and your allergies will be alleviated. While not everyone experiences the same effects, some common beneficial results include:

- Soaring energy and less need to sleep or take a "power nap"
- Better mental clarity, memory, and focus
- Fewer headaches and backaches
- Less arthritis, knee aches, and joint pain
- A reduction in cellulite
- Fewer colds and a stronger immune system
- Fewer symptoms of PMS, hot flashes, night sweats, menopausal symptoms, and other hormone swings

In spite of these benefits, you may be feeling skeptical or even a little intimidated. Most of my clients are surprised to learn that doing the Martha's Vineyard Diet Detox is actually pleasant. You get to enjoy an infinite variety of vegetable soups, fresh veggie juices, and nutritional supplements. Since you create them yourself (following our guidance), you control what they taste like. Partial to Italian flavors or Asian food? No problem. You don't have to deprive yourself of the flavors you love. Concerned about being hungry? Don't worry. You will feed yourself every two hours or less, staving off those uncomfortable hunger pangs. Looking for rapid results? You'll lose weight and see your body change very quickly because you will feed yourself large amounts of nutrients in small doses. As you lose weight, I'm going to encourage you to pay extra attention to your self-care. If you're like most people, you may not know what it looks and feels like to really nurture yourself. I'm going to ask you to take gentle walks, get a few colonics, and journal about the mental, physical, and spiritual sensations you experience as your organs and cells literally unclog themselves. And, because your body naturally balances itself as you engage in the detox, you will no longer experience the cravings that cause many people to pig out and make it difficult to adopt the healthier eating habits they want to incorporate into their lifestyle.

Concerned that you may be too sick to detox? Don't worry. The Martha's Vineyard Diet Detox is very safe. Because it involves consuming maximum nutrition in small doses obtained from food sources, it is very, very healthy to engage in regardless of your physical condition. Of course, it's always important to consult your doctor before making any lifestyle changes, but there is nothing risky about the program. That's definitely not the case with other diets and may not be with other detoxes. Got high cholesterol? No problem. Unlike dieting, which can be dangerous when you're ill, the Martha's Vineyard Diet Detox will give you energy and nutrients rather than make you feel weak or tired. Diabetes? It won't cause your blood sugar to spike or dive. Cancer? It will help strengthen your immune system so your body can naturally fight the disease in ways radiation and chemotherapy cannot. Hypertension? No problem. Many find their blood pressure drops significantly as they clean up their system. Many people enjoy the "miracle" of their body healing itself.

But I'll be honest with you, there's no way around it: You will have to change your lifestyle over the next 21 days—and, hopefully, beyond. For the Martha's Vineyard Diet Detox to work, you will have to chuck the chips, cheeseburgers, cookies, and ice cream. You can't eat processed food while you're on the program. I will clearly explain the lifestyle changes you will need to implement. I've broken everything down into plain English and simple steps to make modifying your lifestyle easier. I'll give you:

- Clear and commonsense examples explaining how this approach works
- Quick-start lifestyle changes, and detoxification and weight-loss techniques that you can begin to implement immediately without reading the entire book
- Comparisons of the Martha's Vineyard Diet Detox with other diets
- Fun quizzes to test your detox savvy
- Answers to questions detoxers frequently ask
- Troubleshooting tips
- Testimonials from real people who participated in the program

Congratulations on committing to making a change. Now let's get going!

Roni DeLuz, RN, ND, PhD
Vineyard Haven, Martha's Vineyard, Massachusetts

Quiz HOW BADLY DO YOU NEED TO DETOX?

Our environment is so polluted that it's impossible to protect yourself from toxins. Still, some of us have been exposed to more noxious substances than others. Take this short quiz and score your results to gain a sense of how toxic a burden your body is carrying.

1. When you think about the environment you live in, would you describe it as: a) very polluted; b) moderately polluted; c) not very polluted at all

2. When you think about the chemicals you use at work and in your home, do you feel that you're exposed: a) a lot; b) very little; c) not at all

3. How would you describe your lifestyle? a) hectic; b) moderately active; c) relaxed

4. Do you suffer indigestion, stomach problems, or frequent gas? a) frequently; b) sometimes; c) never

5. Do you lose energy or get tired during the afternoon? a) yes; b) sometimes; c) never

6. Do you experience food intolerances that give you postnasal drip, blurred vision, burping, headaches, itching, burning eyes, sneezing or swollen eyes, or a swollen face? a) yes, from some specific foods; b) sometimes; c) never

7. Do you have bad breath? a) yes; b) sometimes; c) never

8. Do you experience insomnia? a) yes; b) sometimes; c) never

9. Do you need to pass gas so often that you find yourself in embarrassing situations? a) yes; b) sometimes; c) never

10. Do you have a hard time losing weight? a) yes; b) sometimes; c) never

If you answered at least five of these questions by selecting answer "a," you urgently need to detox. Toxins in your body are significantly compromising your quality of life and may be causing you serious health problems. If letter "b" was your most common choice, noxious substances are lowering your energy level and are probably causing discomforts like headaches and indigestion. You, too, need to detox, but less urgently than some others. Do it at your earliest convenience. If you've chosen letter "c" as your response to most of these questions, consider yourself a lucky and healthy person! Detoxing will give you more energy, get rid of any nagging complaints you may have grown accustomed to, and contribute to your vitality and longevity.

HOW DETOXING SAVED MY LIFE

I didn't set out to become an expert on either weight loss or detoxification. In the spring of 1987, I was an ordinary woman living an ordinary life. I was thirty-two, married, a mother, and happily following my calling as a registered nurse. We lived in Southern California, where my husband and I owned and operated three nursing homes providing health care to medically fragile and developmentally disabled youth. But unbeknownst to my staff and patients, I had begun experiencing medical problems of my own.

In retrospect, my health challenges actually began about two years earlier, when I had started feeling a bit off kilter. I noticed that I was getting occasional headaches that, over time, became more frequent. Since I was very busy at home and at work, I just chalked it up to stress and popped an aspirin. No big deal, I thought. Then, I started feeling a little pain in my joints—nothing too uncomfortable or disabling. I would ignore these indications that something was wrong, down another aspirin or Tylenol, and go on about my life. Little by little, things started getting worse. My joints started aching; my muscles began to hurt; I started having night sweats; my heart started racing.

I sought help, beginning with my internist, who did not know what was wrong and suggested I see another doctor. Over the course of several years, I saw close to thirty physicians: my primary, different neurologists, immunologists, a rheumatoid arthritis expert, several heart specialists, a psychiatrist, a gastroenterologist. None of them could figure out what was going on. Was it lupus? Multiple sclerosis? Cancer? A bone disease? Crohn's disease? A boatload of viruses? Over time, different doctors suspected many ghastly, horrible things, but nobody was certain about what was happening to my body. At first, they told me to keep taking aspirin to relieve my symptoms. Then they started handing me prescriptions: antibiotics, arthritis meds, steroids. At one point I was taking seven different drugs. In the meantime my symptoms kept getting worse and worse—and instead of occurring individually they started happening all at once.

Before long, whatever was going wrong with me took over my body and life. I lost my appetite. I lost weight. I got so constipated that I was only having a bowel movement once every week or two. My thinking became slow and muddled—sometimes my brain was so foggy that it felt like I was stuck in a Coca-Cola bottle and couldn't get out. My body was bloated, my skin hurt, and so did my eyeballs. At one point it felt like bugs were crawling all over me. Needless to say, as my body and life spiraled out of control, I sank into a deep depression.

By 1989, I had basically become bedridden. On one of the rare days that I dragged myself out, I apparently drove in circles for hours while taking my three-year-old daughter Whitney to school. When I snapped out of it, I had no idea where I was, where I'd been, or where the time had gone. That's when I knew something was desperately wrong. I admitted that I had a serious problem. I knew that if I didn't get help, I would be in serious trouble.

You might wonder how someone like me could find myself in a situation like this. As a nurse and a nursing-home owner and administrator, I certainly knew a lot of doctors. I, of all people, should have been able to obtain proper care. So it would seem.

But like many people who develop a chronic illness, I had unknowingly strayed onto what health care providers secretly call "the sick wheel": you go from doctor to doctor to doctor, none of whom knows exactly what's wrong or has the complete picture of what's going on, though each prescribes an additional medicine. When you're on the sick wheel, you end up taking drug after drug after drug—one for the physical symptoms you originally showed up with, then another to cover up the symptoms, or side effects, the first drug causes. After a while your kidneys start hurting from trying to filter the man-made chemicals from the first two drugs out of your system. The kidneys are like the body's trash cans, filtering waste and toxins from the blood, creating urine, and helping to regulate blood pressure, but they aren't designed to process synthetic substances like pharmaceutical drugs. Once they start aching (and if you're on two meds, they eventually will), the doctors typically prescribe a third drug to mask those symptoms. Before long, you have to take a fourth to cover up the symptoms caused by the third one. You reach a point where so many things are going wrong with your body that no one really knows what the problem is: the drugs or the disease.

Many people in the medical community know this cycle by a more ominous name: the "death ceremony." It's only a matter of time before the synthetic ingredients in the drugs wreak havoc inside your body, which becomes burdened with substances it wasn't designed to process and, therefore, experiences as toxic. Eventually, these chemicals exhaust the kidney and liver. Many people end up on dialysis or a transplant list because medicine has damaged their organs. And lots of folks actually die of so-called "side effects" rather than of the disease they're being treated for. In fact, the fourth leading cause of death according to the Food and Drug Administration is cited as "Adverse drug reactions." Not surprisingly, people become depressed as they lose their quality of life and hope. Within medical circles it's a well-known practice that the last drug they give you is Prozac.

Since I worked within the hospital system, I knew I was waltzing a dance with death. I felt lost and alone. My husband, who traveled out of the country on business a fair amount, wasn't always around to support me. When he was there, he looked to *me* for the answers on health matters. Aside from my mother, who would nurture and pray for me, I hid my problems from loved ones. I believed that I was supposed to have all the answers since I was the health practitioner in the family. I knew it was my moral and professional duty to help others, but for some reason, I thought that I wasn't supposed to get sick. Now that I was ill, I felt fearful, ashamed, and isolated, which, of course, made my situation worse.

One of the few people who knew what was going on with me was my girlfriend Deborah Williams. I let Deb talk me into getting a colonic, a holistic health care procedure where a trained practitioner flushes out your colon, or large intestine, with water. The colon is the primary organ that eliminates waste and toxins from the body. When the colon is clean the body is able to purify itself more easily. At the time, hospitals still gave people enemas to clean out their bowels and to help them use the bathroom more easily, so a colonic was nothing but a glorified enema in my mind. Since nothing the doctors were doing was helping and Deb had offered to pay for it, I figured, "Why not?"

During my appointment, colon therapist Eloise Buckner of Agoura, California, explained how the procedure helped remove toxins from the body. (You can learn more about colonics in Chapter 6.) Afterwards, I actually felt a little bit better, although I didn't want to admit it. Still, I let Deb treat me to a second colonic.

"You're overproteinized," Eloise told me.

"Nonsense," I thought to myself. My typical diet consisted of meat and potatoes. "How can you eat too much protein?" I wondered. Yet I had to admit that I felt better after that colonic, too. And she wasn't trying to give me any pills, which was a relief after my previous experiences with medication. Over time, I began to trust Eloise and continued to see her regularly.

Since Deb was right about colonics, I decided to take her advice to go see an herbalist, a health practitioner who treats illness by using plant-based remedies administered as teas, tablets, capsules, and tinctures. The herbalist was shocked to see the list of prescription medications I was taking—and even more surprised that I didn't know why I was on them. The more he asked about my medical treatment, the more I realized I didn't know the answers to some very basic, yet vital, questions. This made me feel both scared and inadequate. I was a nurse, after all! I should have had answers. Prescription drugs, while helpful, are serious business and are not to be taken lightly.

"I know this is going to sound crazy to you," I said, "but my mind is so foggy I feel like I'm in a Coca-Cola bottle."

"You're not crazy, you're sick," he told me. "We're all exposed to many toxins—in the environment, in our homes, and in our workplaces. You're carrying a huge toxic load in your system and your body is being compromised."

That made sense to me. I explained that in my hometown of New Haven, Connecticut, butterflies and ladybugs and little insects were always flying around. But in Thousand Oaks and Simi Valley, California, where I now lived and worked, nothing flew, nothing moved. It was an agricultural area. Crop dusting was prevalent; herbicides and pesticides were ubiquitous. California also has among the nation's most stringent rules involving pest control in nursing facilities. We were always getting sprayed for something.

"Aha! That's the problem: your body can't take this stuff anymore," he told me. "All these drugs you're on are making things worse. We've got to wean you off of them. And your digestive system is very bad. We have to put you on baby food."

The idea of getting off my meds was a big stretch to me. I didn't want to be overmedicated, but at the same time I didn't think it was safe for me to be completely medication free. The thought that I had to eat baby food sounded outrageous. What Dr. Taylor was saying and the way he was thinking were foreign to me, but the more we talked, I sensed that he was right. I felt relieved and hopeful for the first time.

For several months baby food was my only form of sustenance. I lost a lot of weight, which concerned me since I was already small because I was sick. My herbalist just told me that if I wanted to maintain my weight to eat more of it. I wasn't exactly in love with the stuff and it's hard to eat 20 jars of baby food every day, but I ate enough to sustain me. Before long I noticed my energy returning. In about three months, I felt noticeably better. And I had started moving my bowels more often, which I knew was an important sign.

Today, I understand that my body was releasing a boatload of toxins. That organic baby food was pure (no artificial flavors, colors, or preservatives) and simple enough (just pure fruit or vegetable with nothing else mixed in) that a baby's newly formed digestive system could tolerate it. It was a lot easier for my body to break down than regular food, healthier than the food I'd been eating, and it allowed my digestive system to rest. As my body grew stronger, one by one the herbalist began weaning me off of prescription drugs.

Feeling better and slowly recovering my life, something told me to order a copy of my medical chart. When it arrived, it was huge! I read every page of notes each of the doctors had written from all my appointments over the years. Toward the end of my file, I came across one set of notations called SOAP (an acronym for *subjective, objective, assessment, plan*) notes, in which the doctor or nurse assesses and summarizes what is going on with the patient, then writes a plan for their care. Here's what my SOAP notes said:

Subjective: "Feeling weak, feverish, my joints ache, and I have a severe headache; I feel like I am in a Coke bottle and I can't get out."
Objective: Well dressed and well-informed female presenting in office once again with multiple symptoms.
Assessment: Temperature: 99.2; Pulse: 88; Respiration: 20; Blood pressure: 98/60; Weight: 128 lbs; Skin: warm, dry; Affect: flat.
Plan: Prozac 40 mg QD, RTC in 90 days.

The word hit me like a ton of bricks: *Prozac,* the death ceremony. The doctors had placed me in it. I felt like I was being stabbed in the heart. My medical peers had given up and written me off, as I'd seen happen to many other patients.

"My God! If I don't save my life, no one will save it for me," I realized.

From that point on—even though I was still a registered nurse—I lost faith in my medical peers' ability to help me get well. I had no idea what I was going to do, but I realized that I had to go on a rampage to save my own life.

By this time my marriage had fallen apart and I was a single mother. I was desperate, scared, and slowly losing my business. My childhood friend, Tony DeLuz, came to California, rescued me, and became my business partner and husband. Tony helped me hold on to my business, which allowed me to focus on getting better.

After about a year of working with Eloise and my herbalist, one of them told me about a clinic in Mexico that offered treatments you couldn't obtain in the United States. Deb and I went there for about two weeks, while Tony and my staff held down the fort.

At the American Biologics Clinic in Tijuana, Mexico, health care was approached very differently than in the United States. Instead of prescribing medications, the clinic used natural remedies to improve my immune function, thereby allowing my own body to fight the toxins and viruses invading it. I tested positive for a few latent viruses that live dormant in your cells, including cytomegalovirus (CMV), which they explained was compromising my liver, as well as chronic fatigue syndrome (CFS) and fibromyalgia, neither of which I had heard of. CFS is characterized by devastating tiredness that prohibits you from performing common activities. Fibromyalgia affects the muscles and joints and the endocrine and cognitive systems, causing anxiety, chronic pain, apathy, confusion and irritability.

Years later, I would identify myself as having environmental illness (EI), where exposure to environmental hazards like chemicals, allergens, pollution, and other toxins makes you sick or aggravates existing medical conditions.

All these conditions are common among people whose bodies are overloaded with toxic chemicals, but at that time American medical professionals were just learning about them. If you were experiencing their symptoms, most doctors would tell you that it was "all in your head," when, in fact, they require a multispecialist approach since they affect so many different organs and systems. In Mexico, I received many different treatments that I hadn't known about before—live-blood-cell therapy, intravenous vitamin drips, coffee enemas—and, yes, more colonics. I was stunned to discover that there were many more ways to help people heal than I had been exposed to in the United States. When I left Mexico, I was still very sick but I felt hopeful, noticeably better, and was able to begin working again.

Once I returned home, I threw myself into learning everything I could about holistic medicine. I was still ill so I did most of my studying in bed. By now, I knew that a healthy colon would be the key to my recovery, so I studied to become certified as a colon therapist, earning my certificate in 1993. Around that time Tony and I relocated back to Connecticut. I returned to nursing, practicing, among other places, at Yale–New Haven Hospital.

As I studied natural healing, I began to learn that alternative doctors are preventing heart attacks and minimizing the need for prescription drugs and surgery by doing things like helping people eat healthier foods, strengthening their immune systems, and administering treatments designed to remove poisonous heavy metals like arsenic and mercury from their body. The more I learned, the more I grew disenchanted—and sometimes even angry—with my profession. While complementary medicine, a diverse collection of health care practices and products that fall outside of the traditions of conventional medicine, isn't the end all and be all, it does have a lot to offer. Unfortunately, the medical establishment looks down on it.

I earned my PhD in natural healing in 1996. Thirsty for more knowledge, I enrolled in the Clayton School of Natural Healing to receive my ND (naturopathic doctor degree). A naturopath differs from a traditional allopathic doctor educated at a typical American medical school. Allopathic physicians are trained to diagnose and treat diseases, prescribe drugs, and perform invasive surgical procedures. They do not learn much about prevention, how a person can heal his or her own body, or how to correct the root causes or reasons a person developed a health condition in the first place, though few will just come out and tell you this.

Naturopaths are trained to be both healers and educators. We believe that, when provided with the right conditions, the body naturally and innately heals itself. Our job is to teach our clients how to create those conditions. A naturopath's training is similar to that of an allopathic doctor, but instead of learning how to prescribe drugs and perform surgery (which we believe are useful, but just not the treatment of first choice), we are trained to treat our clients with foods, nutritional supplements, herbs, enemas, colonics, various mind/body/spirit approaches, iridology, Chinese medicine, Ayurvedic medicine (a healing system native to India), and stress reduction and relaxation techniques that help the body heal itself.

In naturopathic school I learned many important concepts that would help me to heal myself. For example, that brain fog/Coke bottle feeling that caused me to feel "out of it" and unable to find my daughter's school? I learned it's a classic symptom of *Candida*, a type of fungus, wherein the body is overrun with yeast cells, and that you can get rid of it by going on an anti-*Candida* cleanse and strict program of dietary changes, herbs, and phytonutrients.

I also realized that I had to be able to understand and help people who were sick access their mind–body connection. So I next studied and became certified as a hypnotist by the American Institute of Hypnotherapy. Knowing hypnosis also helped me overcome my own physical challenges. As I educated myself, I "test drove" on my own body every procedure I learned in school. I learned their strengths and limitations, what worked and what didn't. Overall, I was amazed by the results!

One day, I woke up and realized I felt great. I had the kind of feeling that makes you sing in the shower at the top of your lungs! I don't know what happened on that particular morning; wellness is a process, it doesn't come in a magic pill. Yet I've learned that there's often a point at which you get over some kind of hump and suddenly realize you're getting better. It had taken me seven years, but I accomplished my goal of healing myself!

While I was engaged in this exhausting process of studying and healing, my old friend Deb told me about Martha's Vineyard, Massachusetts. Though I had grown up in and lived in Connecticut, about four hours from "The Vineyard," as the island is called, I didn't know anything about this playground for the "rich and famous." I hadn't had any downtime since I could remember, so I gladly investigated. The ferry ride over was beautiful. I felt rejuvenated by the blue skies, the feel of warm sunshine on my face, the seagulls that waft alongside the boat as it travels, and the smell of the fresh sea air. When I arrived, I felt like I was in heaven. I loved the pastel-colored gingerbread cottages, the dramatic cliffs, the island's scenic lighthouses. I decided that I had to live there. Within a year my family and I had moved into a spacious home in the town of Oak Bluffs.

I worked as a nurse at Windemere Nursing and Rehabilitation Center. I had mixed feelings about being back in a hospital setting, but my return to traditional medicine taught me a lot. I found that I felt guilty distributing the roughly twenty-five pills I provided to many of my patients daily, knowing that I was exposing them to the medicines' side effects. I realized, instead, that I wanted to teach people to repair, regenerate and rejuvenate themselves by detoxifying their bodies. As a side job, I began working with older people who were interested in being weaned off of medications. Over time, my client list grew. I also started a support group for people with CFS. Word traveled that I knew how to help people heal. Before long, my house was filled with friends and guests wanting me to help them get better from CFS, cancer, diabetes, multiple sclerosis. I did.

In the middle of all this, I bore my son Toron. I also have an older stepson, Tony, Jr., who is older than my daughter Whitney. My pregnancy put more stress on my healing-but-still-fragile body than it was able to handle. After giving birth, it took me a month to walk and two years to recover. While nursing myself back to optimal health, I developed the cleansing program and healing philosophy behind the Martha's Vineyard Diet Detox. I was able to resume a full life as a wife, mother, and healer, so I knew it could work for others.

In 1999 I opened the Martha's Vineyard Holistic Retreat (www.mvholisticretreat.com), located at the Martha's Vineyard Inn in Vineyard Haven. My background allows me to integrate traditional Western and alternative approaches, while my experience in acute and chronic care allows me to help people who are extremely sick. My clients range from islanders to vacationers to New Age gurus to medical doctors, some of whom say they fear being run out of their profession for pursuing alternative care. In the off-season I travel around the country and treat people in their homes.

I noticed that as I detoxed my clients to help them improve their health, they would feel thrilled that they were also losing weight. I kept reminding them that they were healing from chronic diseases, but they kept talking about dropping pounds. In time, I started to understand just how important weight loss was to them. Indeed, a healthy body and a healthy weight go hand in hand, and weight loss is a wonderful consequence of detoxifying the body. But between the demands of starting a business, beginning menopause (at which point my metabolism slowed to a crawl), and not exercising, I started to get quite heavy. Although I was eating very healthy foods, over several years I gained about 50 pounds. This really bothered me. Even prior to getting sick, I had been obsessed with dieting. Weight has always been a challenge for me; the women in my family tend to be hippy and we all carry weight around our butts. Over the years I'd done a lot of research on diets and dieting and tried them all: Atkins, Pritikin, high protein, low carb. None of them worked. Fortunately, by this time I knew that toxicity must play a role, but I was so busy helping to heal others that I didn't address my own weight problem right away.

One day James Hester, an entertainment industry marketing and promotions professional, came to stay at the Inn. He was surprised not only by how much younger and vibrant he looked after detoxing, but by how both his energy level and outlook on life improved during the process. I detoxed James twice. He lost 21 pounds each time. (You can read James's testimonial on page 16.) He started referring his friends and family. They detoxed, lost weight, felt better, and looked great. But after he knew me fairly well, James got on my case, insisting that I needed to lose weight. At his urging I decided to heed my own advice and lost the 50 pounds. My metabolism is still extremely slow, but I keep my weight down by following the program. In the meantime James kept referring people to me. Each time, he observed that everyone lost weight.

"This detoxing for health is great," he told me. "But I am convinced that you have a diet—a detox diet!" He went on a mission to get me this book deal. In order to prove that my program worked. I detoxed my publisher Judith Regan, who lost 21 pounds. My cowriter, Hilary Beard, also detoxed but, like many people, didn't want to lose weight. You can read her story on page 185 and tips for detoxing while maintaining your size in Chapter 8.

Testimonial
JAMES HESTER

I'm no newcomer to dieting. In the course of my career as a publicist in the entertainment industry, I've worked with a slew of actors, models, and singers. Because I work very closely with my clients, I've tried all kinds of diets, nutritionists, chefs, and trainers with them. Each time, by the end of each week of not being able to eat what I wanted and doing squats and working out until my legs were aching and burning, I'd only lose about 3 or 4 pounds—in part because I had to attend a lot of premieres and dinner parties. Still, it was a lot of pain for very little gain.

In 2002, I experienced a personal and professional betrayal when I was let go from my job. After seventeen years in the entertainment industry, I found myself out of work. I was furious! I was probably the angriest I have been in my entire life. I put my furniture in storage and took some time off to visit family and friends. Like most people, I used food as a crutch to help me manage my emotions. I ate and ate and ate. I consider my ideal weight to be 175 to 180 pounds—185 max. But in January 2003, I was the fattest I'd ever been in my life: carrying 213 pounds on my 5-foot, 10-inch frame. I had a huge stomach, I was getting fat folds on my back, I had a double-going-on-triple chin, and my skin was bumpy and blotchy. I couldn't zip up my pants but I refused to buy a larger size; I wore big shirts instead. I didn't feel good mentally or spiritually. I knew I had to get control of myself.

I asked a number of my friends if they knew of a healing spa or retreat. One of my friends referred me to a facility in Mexico. I went there for a while and went on a diet that included a lot of grilled salmon, steamed vegetables, rolled oats, almond milk, bananas, fruit, and lots of water and ozone. I stayed away from white flour and sugar about 85 percent of the time. I lost 10 pounds, which left me at 203. I stayed on this diet until about the end of March. At that point I planned to stay with some friends in southern Florida for a few weeks until I found housing. I figured I would live there for a while, continue my healthy lifestyle, and get some more of this weight off. I had everything organized and planned.

About five days before I was going to leave for Florida, I was talking on the phone to a friend whose house I would be staying at, when she clicked over to take another call. When she got back on the line, she told me, "Deborah Williams says hello."

Deborah Williams is the sister-in-law of the famous publicist Marvet Britto. Marvet had referred me to the doctor I visited in Mexico. Deborah was the person who had told Marvet about it, so I called Deborah to thank her.

"Oh, I'm so glad you went!" Deborah told me. I told her that my stay there had gone well and that in a couple of days I'd be starting a new regime at my friend's place in South Florida. "I'm going to walk and do yoga and take wheatgrass juice," I told her. "But I wish there was one place I could go where I could do everything under one roof so I wouldn't have to figure out what to do, where to go, and who to see for myself."

"Well, my best friend has a retreat in Martha's Vineyard," she told me. "I grew up and went to college with her. She is an amazing woman. Her name's Dr. Roni DeLuz."

"Martha's Vineyard? Last summer I took the ferry over there for a quick lunch in Edgartown. I loved the feel of the place! Give me her number, please. I'll cancel all this stuff I was planning to do on my own if I can get that kind of support."

So Deborah gave me her number and I called Dr. DeLuz.

"It's off-season," Dr. DeLuz told me. "We're really not open now."

"I want to come now," I persisted. I didn't know who this woman was or what her credentials were, but for some reason it felt like that's where I needed to go. I didn't realize it at the time because I wasn't active spiritually, but the inner God in me was leading me, and the God in me was trusting.

With much persistence on my part, she finally relented.

With that I canceled all the arrangements and appointments I had set up in Florida. My family thought I was nuts. "You don't even know where you're going," they told me.

"I don't care. I'm going."

For the next 3 days, I proceeded to gorge myself. I ate everything I wanted. Once I arrived on the Vineyard on Sunday, April 13, I dropped off my stuff at the Inn. I walked around the town of Vineyard Haven eating anything I could get my hands on: a bagel, pizza, ice cream, a pound of chocolate. I ate until I was sick, but I was determined that the next morning I would continue eating like I had in Mexico: grilled fish, steamed vegetables, steamed broccoli, lots of water, no sugars, and so on.

On the morning of Monday, April 14, 2003, I had my first meeting with Dr. Roni DeLuz. "I really want to get healthy," I told her. "I want to eat steamed fish, vegetables, oatmeal, blah, blah, blah."

Roni started shaking her head.

"Come over here," she told me, leading me to a chalkboard in the dining room. "At 8:00 you'll have what's called MetaBerries; then at 10:00 you'll have this supplement; at noon you'll have live fresh vegetable juice consisting of carrots, ginger, or whatever . . ." She ran down the line-up of what I would eat, but none of it was anything I recognized as food.

"Yeah, but you don't understand," I told her. "I want to lose weight, but I want to eat grilled fish and I don't want to have to go into town to get it."

"No, no, no," she insisted. "This is what you'll be eating all day."

"Wait a minute! You're telling me this is what I'm going to eat for the whole time I'm here?! Where are my steamed vegetables? I want to eat healthy."

"This is healthier than you'll ever eat."

On the inside, I was like, "Yeah, right, you *freak!*" On the outside I said, "But I want to lose weight."

"You'll lose 21 pounds if you're here for 21 days. Is that a problem?" Twenty-one pounds would get me down to 182—the weight I wanted to be. But it wasn't worth being hungry.

"If that's all I eat, I'm going to starve!" I protested.

"No, James, you won't be hungry at all."

"Wait a minute! You're telling me that if I do everything you just went through on this board, I'm never going to be hungry and I'm going to walk out of here 21 pounds lighter?"

"Is that a problem?"

"If you help me lose 21 pounds in 21 days, I'll spread the word to everyone I know and get you a book deal!"

"Well, you *are* going to lose 21 pounds, and I would *love* to have a book deal. But my main goal is to get you healthy."

"Well, let's go!"

Dr. Roni had definitely gotten my attention, but to tell you the truth, I thought she was crazy. I'd worked with supermodel Beverly Johnson for years. I knew what she went through to get herself ready for a big photo shoot—all those squats and lunges and being hungry all the time. It was rough, even with personal chefs and trainers. All those diets were a big sacrifice. And I never lost 21 pounds in 21 days! Now, here was this woman I didn't know saying that I could lose that much weight without being hungry. I was definitely down to try it.

On that first day I was all gung-ho. I wanted it and everyone I met at the Inn seemed so nice. But being the control freak that I was at the time (and somewhat still am), I wasn't 100 percent trusting. I kept trying to run the show. I didn't even know what I was running, but I was trying to run it! Even so, I was diligent and heeded Dr. Roni's advice to stick to her schedule of receiving nutrients every two hours. She said I wouldn't feel hungry if I did this; if I didn't, I was at risk of going into the danger zone where I might pig out on the first thing in sight. I didn't want to be hungry, and I didn't want to blow my chances at that kind of weight loss, so I stayed on schedule.

But while I was learning to control my eating, I began to realize that I was still an extremely angry person. At the retreat, I would tell my story to anyone who would listen to me. "She did this to me. Blah, blah, blah. . . ." Everyone who treated me—the colon therapist, the masseuse, the homeopathic psychotherapist, everyone who would listen—heard my story over and over. "Blah, blah, blah. . . ." I didn't know anything about detoxing at the time. I now realize that as you're cleansing your body, you're also cleaning up your emotions. For days as I detoxed, I purged my anger and the sense of betrayal I had been carrying around.

On Day 3 I experienced what I now know is a "healing crisis," the reaction you have as the body flushes toxins out of your cells so you can excrete them in your urine and bowel movements. In my case, it manifested itself in constantly feeling cold. Then twelve to fourteen hours later—just as quickly as it began—it ended. That was the worst thing that happened to me during the 21 days. I got colonics, which I had received before, and coffee enemas, which I'd never experienced, and did everything they told me to do.

Three days later I was feeling really good. Things were starting to roll; I was experiencing physical and mental changes. And for the first time in my life I enjoyed spending time alone. I started realizing that I actually liked myself! I took daily walks past the Vineyard's restaurants and smelled the wonderful fragrances floating out of them, but I didn't crave anything. I wasn't tempted at all! I was so excited about what I was experiencing that I wanted to stay on the program. Mentally, I realized I was also shedding toxic emotions. I felt like a million bucks and also started thinking, "The world needs to know about this Diet Detox."

On one of my walks I had seen a church right down the street from the Inn. I realized it was almost Easter. I asked one of the women who worked at the Inn if she was going to church. She told me she wasn't going to go to church; she'd be taking care of me. I had grown up a devout Catholic. In my family, Easter Sunday had been a big deal. I couldn't believe that this woman who I knew had two children was going to be with me instead of her two kids! As I talked to the other staff at the retreat, I learned that she wasn't the only one making this sacrifice to take care of me. I couldn't believe it! I went into town and bought everything chocolate in sight—Easter bunnies, Easter eggs, chocolate-coated marshmallow bunnies, all kinds of Easter candy. At the supermarket one of the staff members saw me with all these sweets. She got a pained look on her face.

"Don't ask any questions," I told her. "It's all right."

"But you're doing so well, James. You should really stay healthy."

"Everything's all right." I took all this candy back to the Inn and closed myself in my room. Every now and then someone would knock on my door.

"Are you okay in there?"

"I'm fine."

I would come out of my room and everyone would be looking at me.

"How are you?"

"I'm fine."

Later that day I gave all the women big Easter baskets for their children and all the people in their lives I knew were making a sacrifice because they would be caring for me. They couldn't believe what I had done. I hadn't been tempted by the candy at all!

That night I pulled Roni aside and gave her some very high-quality soaps. "Please accept this gift," I told her. "Tomorrow is Easter Sunday. I feel really grateful to God for what He's doing for me."

"That's what will happen if you let it happen," she told me, and explained that detoxing is the perfect time to really cleanse your spirit.

"I have to go to church tomorrow," I told her. I knew Dr. Roni would be going to church the next day and asked if I could join her.

The pastor's sermon that morning was very interesting but I have to admit I don't remember what she said—the service ran late and I started getting hungry. I knew I had to have my next supplement soon or I was going to "crash." Before the service ended, the pastor told the congregation that she was going to baptize a young lady. Dr. Roni knew we were already running late, so she told me that as the family walked to the front of the church we could sneak out quietly. Then the pastor asked if anyone else wanted to be baptized. Out of nowhere, Spirit grabbed hold of me. I stood up and said, "I want to be baptized." Dr. Roni looked at me and said, "Really?!" The people in the church shouted, "Hallelujah! Amen!"

I had no idea what I was doing, but the next thing I knew two men took me into a side room and put me in a robe. Before she baptized us, the pastor said we'd be filled with the Holy Ghost and God would forgive all our sins—they would be washed away by the water. I went down in the water in Jesus's name. When I came up, I was baptized. That's when things really started working in my life.

On the way home Dr. Roni stopped by a house. She told me she owned it and was preparing to rent it for the summer. It had a big living room and a big loft. It occurred to me that my furniture would fit perfectly in the space. I was homeless by choice because I hadn't figured out what I was going to do with my life. All of my things were in storage. We made arrangements for me to rent the house for four months.

By Day 10 of my detox I couldn't believe what was happening to me. I was losing tons of weight and was feeling great! My pores had cleaned themselves out. And my double chin was gone! It looked like I had had a facelift! Emotionally, I felt amazing. And I was reconnecting with my spirit. I was letting God come in and clean me out.

The last week of the detox continued successfully. I could not believe that I wasn't chewing but wasn't starving and thinking, "Oh, God, I want a hamburger! I just have to have a bite of cheesecake." I'd walk by people eating all of those things and wouldn't even think about it.

By Day 21 I had lost 21 pounds. When I had arrived at the Inn my clothes had been too tight; now everything except my sweatpants with the elastic waist was falling off of me. Suddenly, I had a great body—I looked and felt like a teenager! I had tons and tons of energy. I had never been a lazy person; I had worked long days my whole adult life. But when my workday was over, I wasn't the type who would exercise. For recreation, I'd drag myself to the movies. In retrospect, I am now able to see that even though I had a wonderful life, I was about 10 percent grateful to God and 90 percent negative, negative, negative—which leaves you completely exhausted.

After completing the 21 days, I looked like a totally different person—and I was one. They held a little ceremony for me on that final day, celebrating the fact that a new life had been born in me on many levels. Dr. Roni told me I had completed the first level of detoxification, and that as I continued to take care of myself, I'd go to higher and higher levels. She was right; I still have issues but I feel and behave so differently. I continue to work on improving my eating habits and my outlook on life, making strides toward becoming a better, healthier person. Because of the Martha's Vineyard Diet Detox, I have undergone a physical, mental, and spiritual transformation. I live my life by Dr. Roni's theory: 75 percent clean and healthy, 25 percent recreational.

1

TOXIC, UNHEALTHY, AND HEAVY
America's Rude Awakening

The United States has the best health care system in the world, yet Americans of all backgrounds are having a hard time staying healthy. At least 20 million Americans are chronically ill with conditions that undermine their quality of life and may ultimately lead to their demise—diseases like cancer, diabetes, heart disease, high cholesterol, hypertension, and kidney and liver failure. Each week, about 80 percent of adults take medication—at least one-third of us down five different drugs—the Institute of Medicine reports. Often, the conditions these medicines treat are caused by our lack of success in maintaining a healthy weight.

Today, over 60 percent of Americans weigh more than their recommended body mass index (BMI), which measures the amount of body fat we carry compared to our height. Sixty-two percent of women and 70 percent of men are overweight, meaning that their BMI is 25 or more (normal is 18.5 to 24.9). Thirty-one percent of men and women are obese. Of course, everyone has different advice for how to slim down. These days, it's almost impossible to figure out whether to eat or avoid carbohydrates; how much protein to consume; whether butter or margarine is better; if fat free also means low calorie; whether foods like red wine, chocolate, and coffee are healthy after all; or if we should sign up for Jenny Craig, Weight Watchers, or L.A. Weight Loss. The advice seems to change almost daily.

Most experts tell us that whether we gain or lose weight is determined by the number of calories we eat compared to the number of calories we burn. If we want to lose weight, we should consume fewer calories, increase our activity level, or, better yet, do both. But while many Americans try to take weight off, experts now know that traditional weight-reduction dieting does not work. Fewer than 5 percent of dieters succeed in keeping the weight they lost off for five years, according to the National Association to Advance Fat Acceptance. A stunning 90 percent of people gain some or all of their weight back, and one-third end up weighing more.

I certainly believe in eating healthy amounts of food and becoming more active, but my experience as a patient, researcher, and healer makes it clear to me that the explanations and approaches toward weight loss based on this approach are incomplete. Scientists are now learning that losing weight is much more complicated than merely balancing calories eaten and burned. We now know that factors as wide ranging as whether we skip breakfast, eat enough healthy foods, get sufficient sleep, have a metabolic disorder, or suffer from intestinal parasites are also part of the equation. These factors and other emerging research on factors affecting weight gain all speak to the importance of living a healthy lifestyle.

The Trouble with Toxins

One of the most significant but least-talked-about factors affecting each individual's weight is the amount of exposure they've had to toxic substances. Noxious materials we encounter in our environment, home, workplace, and food supply are altering our bodies in fundamental and detrimental ways. Of course, everyone knows that certain toxins make us sick. Who isn't aware that cigarette smoke can cause heart disease and cancer—and, as we're now learning, not just in the smoker but also among those who inhale the secondhand fumes? We know that lead poisoning can cause learning disabilities, behavioral problems, and a lower IQ, among other problems. Researchers have recently identified both cigarette smoke and lead as causing one-third of attention deficit hyperactivity disorder (ADHD) cases. Mercury now contaminates large predatory fish like shark, albacore tuna, and mackerel. And toxins like dioxin are not only ubiquitous but a major cause of cancer.

But who knew that poisons like these could mess up our metabolism? Gaining weight is one common but little-known and poorly understood consequence of body processes gone haywire in the presence of poisonous substances. The damage toxins inflict upon us can make it exceedingly difficult—if not impossible—for some people to shed excess pounds. Now don't get me wrong; of course, it's true that many dieters fail because they exercise poor portion control—or don't exercise their bodies at all. But I can't tell you how many people I've worked with who eat surprisingly little, healthy food, yet can barely shed a pound. Lots of people approach weight loss diligently; yet few have long-lasting results. Many repeat dieters sense that something's wrong—for example, they know that their results do not reflect their effort—but since our culture places the responsibility for being overweight on the individual, they wrongly blame themselves for their lack of success. But I'm here to tell you that even if you do sometimes lack self-discipline, and even if you don't always stick to your weight-loss program to the letter, *the fact that you're fat may not be your fault!* You may be a victim of toxins.

Fortunately, we can all take steps to reduce our body's toxic load. Detoxifying our bodies can help us improve our health—including preventing, controlling, and even healing from chronic and life-altering diseases like high cholesterol, hypertension, and diabetes. As it detoxifies, the body sheds excess weight. In this book you will learn how to lose weight in a way that helps you keep unwanted pounds off and helps you transition into the healthier lifestyle you may have desired.

Since you're reading this book, I probably don't need to warn you about the dangers of factory smoke or tell you to go inside when the truck spraying insecticide drives through your neighborhood. But not all the toxins we are exposed to are delivered in a way that is so obvious. In fact, most noxious ingredients appear to be so harmless that we have them in our homes, use them on our bodies, and even eat them every day. Ever wonder why you can't stand the smell of bleach? Why you are supposed to paint only in a well-ventilated room? Why you aren't supposed to get weed killer on your hands? Because they contain ingredients that the body can't tolerate.

Surprisingly, our water supply contains the chemical fluoride, one of the most ubiquitous toxic substances. Fluoride helps prevent tooth decay; yet, research has also linked it to bone cancer, lower IQs, and osteoporosis. As evidenced by a feature story in *Prevention* magazine,[1] increasing numbers of people believe that fluoride should be removed from our water. Personal care products ranging from antiperspirant to hair coloring to nail polish also contain toxic substances. But don't believe me; read the fine print on the packages. (Better yet, Google the ingredients so you can learn more about them.) Most brands of toothpaste, a product we put in our mouths at least twice daily for our entire lives, contain sodium laurel sulfate to make it foam, but which research shows can damages the immune system and can cause inflammation. Many toothpastes also contain fluoride. There is actually a warning on the box to call poison control if your child swallows too much of it. These days, beauty experts recommend that we use bronzing products to obtain a sun-kissed glow without exposing ourselves unnecessarily to dangerous ultraviolet rays. So I was surprised to get a call about a news story on Boston's CBS television affiliate stating that beauty salon spray-on tans contain mercury, lead, and even arsenic. The website of the Food and Drug Administration (FDA; www.fda.gov)—the organization charged with protecting the public health by ensuring the safety of our food supply, drugs, cosmetics, and other substances—says this about them: "Consumers should request measures to protect their eyes and mucous membranes and prevent inhalation." If that doesn't

---

[1] Timothy Gower, "The Danger in Your Water," *Prevention*, August 2006.

indicate that the procedure, which is entirely legal, is also toxic, I don't know what does.

Since you probably have drunk tap water for much of your life and have yet to drop dead of fluoride poisoning, you may be feeling skeptical and wondering how I define the word *toxic*. Plain and simple: *The body experiences as noxious any substance it doesn't know how to process into food or eliminate as waste.* If its ingredients cannot be used as fuel or be purged through sweat, feces, or urine, it is incompatible with the body. Sherry A. Rogers, MD, of Syracuse, New York, one of the world's leading experts in environmental medicine (the relationship between illness and the environment), states in her book *Detoxify or Die*: "Toxins are not normal to the body, they are not meant to be metabolized by the body, and we do not have the metabolic machinery to completely detoxify them."[2] What makes these ingredients incompatible with our bodies is that our cells don't know what to do with them.

The implications of a substance's not being "normal" to our bodies or of its not knowing what to do with it are very far reaching. As we learned in high school biology class, the body evolved over tens of thousands of years. Our organs and systems are amazingly well equipped to process substances our forbears have eaten or contacted for generations. They have a harder time dealing with ingredients they have had little experience dealing with. So unless your ancestors have been eating or using it forever, the less a substance resembles the animal, vegetable, or mineral source it was derived from, the less compatible it is with your body.

This exposure factor becomes a big problem when you live in a world that is changing quickly—and in a society that thrives on innovation, as ours does. New products or ingredients may improve our quality of life, but if our bodies aren't familiar with them, they need time to adapt. When I observe how quickly our children learn their way around the computer or how easily they multitask when compared to their parents, it's clear that the brain is keeping up with the rapid pace of change. The body, on the other hand,

---

[2] Sherry A. Rogers, *Detoxify or Die* (Syracuse, NY: Prestige Publishing, 2002).

is lagging behind, which is one reason why we're becoming heavy and sick. When exposed to a substance it is unfamiliar with, the body does not have the tools or processes it needs to metabolize or eliminate it. Consequently, it will have an allergic reaction (the body's way of rejecting and attempting to expel it), or it will store the substance because it doesn't know what to do with it.

Because noxious substances often aren't accompanied by an ominous-looking cloud or pungent odor or even a skull-and-crossbones label, most of us are unaware of the number of toxic items we encounter each day. As a result, we don't take precautions to avoid or protect ourselves from them. Nor do we know how to purge them from our system. For instance, in addition to fluoride, tap water often contains lead residue from old pipes and prescription drugs other people throw down the drain but that the water-filtration system does not remove. These are toxic. Even if you try to avoid tap-water toxins by drinking bottled water, the plastic bottles the water comes in contain noxious ingredients called phthalates. Such toxins are so common that they are "totally unavoidable," writes Dr. Rogers. She states that biopsy studies performed by the Environmental Protection Agency (EPA) "show that 100% of people had dioxins, PCBs, dichlorobenzene, and xylem." Research shows that dioxins and PCBs (polychlorinated biphenyls) are among the most dangerous carcinogens known to man. Hazardous chemicals like them are so ubiquitous, she writes, that they can even be found in the breast milk of Inuit women living in the Arctic Circle.

A 2005 study published by the Environmental Working Group (EWG), an environmental watchdog group composed of professionals from many disciplines, supports Dr. Rogers's claims. Researchers for the EWG tested the umbilical cord blood of ten newborns for the presence of toxins and discovered 287 different chemicals circulating in their blood supply. These ranged from pesticides to consumer product ingredients to wastes from burning coal, gas, and garbage. Of them, 180 have been proven to cause cancer, 217 poison the brain and nervous system, and 208 cause birth defects or abnormal development in animals.

Over time, dangerous chemicals like these accumulate in our

cells, creating what scientists call the body's *toxic load* or *toxic burden*. As our toxic load increases, we often feel "off" but may become used to it, or, as I did, get in the habit of popping a pill. Unless we make changes to reduce our toxic burden, our symptoms inevitably worsen. After several decades during which they "wreak havoc with our hormones and accelerate the aging process," they "eventually produce disease," Dr. Rogers writes. Consistent with her assertions, public health experts now tell us that 95 percent of cancers as well as most diseases are caused by the environment and diet. The EWG study notes that "scientists cannot fully explain" rising rates of many health disorders—from a tenfold increase in childhood autism rates, to a doubling of birth defects among baby boys, to a 40 percent increase in brain cancer among kids, to a 23 percent increase in premature births. However, "early life exposure to environmental pollutants is a leading suspect," the researchers state.

As people begin to learn about the dangers common substances pose, a common response is to become angry or disheartened because the government doesn't protect us from them. The government actually does protect us—but there are limits. For example, the FDA examines the ingredients found in food, drugs, and cosmetics. Most of the ingredients the agency approves, while not always completely healthy, aren't that bad for us. We all know that if, for example, we rinse with mouthwash—some brands contain roughly 25 percent alcohol, which is noxious—we're not going to keel over. But each time we come in contact with a toxic substance, a little of it stays in us because the body does not know how to get rid of it. And the FDA only tests these substances' toxic effect individually. Nobody—not consumers, not the product manufacturers, and not the government—has any idea what happens when we use hundreds of these products every day for the rest of our lives, as all of us do. Of course, it's impossible to test an individual's exposure to everything, every day, forever—especially when new products are being introduced daily.

But there's a darker side to the story. Many experts believe that our elected officials and government agencies have been bought out by big business. Dr. Rogers writes: "Industry relies on people being too busy, too tired, too sick, and too disinterested in taking responsibility for their health to ever take the time to learn these facts, much less do anything about them." And let's be honest: if the government were to take on every toxic product, there would be tremendous negative consequences to the economy—and to American jobs!

Food for Thought

Americans' unhealthy relationship with food also causes us to gain weight. First of all, we eat too much. From twenty-four-hour grocery stores to fast-food restaurants at every major intersection, to snack foods at the gas station mini-market, food is at our fingertips, twenty-four hours a day, seven days a week. At midnight, we can run to the drive-through and order a quarter-pound cheeseburger, super-sized fries, and a sixty-four-ounce soda. During one movie, it's common for a person to down a tub of salty, buttery popcorn that just a few years ago would have been considered large enough to feed a family. We're served a huge bowl of salad, croutons, and dressing and endless garlic-butter bread sticks at the local Italian food chain—and that's before we get to our oversized course of pasta. Because enormous amounts of food are pervasive in our society, we take it for granted that this is how things should be. But travel to another country and you quickly discover not only that things are different there but just how out of line we are. No other society in the history of humankind has been so oversaturated with food. Given the incredible level of excess we experience, it's no wonder that few of us can resist the temptations.

On top of that, what many of us eat is not very good for us. Our supermarkets and takeout, sit-down, and fast-food restaurants are filled with foods that are high in fat, cholesterol, sodium, artificial flavors and colors, hormones, and preservatives. To make groceries last longer on supermarket shelves, manufacturers strip foods of important nutrients and then "enrich" them with man-made vitamins and minerals. But the body cannot process man-made ingredients as effectively as the "real thing." Because the body doesn't know what to do with any of these synthetic additives, they accumulate inside us as toxins.

What's more, most of us don't consume enough nutrients. We may not be starving for food like the emaciated people living in famine zones we see on the nightly news, but we are definitely malnourished. Our dietary deficiencies manifest themselves as "thunder thighs," "beer bellies," "cottage cheese behind," "baby weight," "middle-age spread" and upper arms that keep waving goodbye long after your guests are gone. And let's not forget being "model thin"; you can fit our cultural standard of beauty and still be very unhealthy.

In fact, even though we're often called the "land of plenty," the average American consumes so few nutrients that they will not be able to live a full life and stay well until they die. Poor nutrition is a major reason that so many of us gain weight, lose energy, and end up on the couch at night in front of the television. It's why we are too tired to ride bikes with our children, take classes at night to change our career, or jog to wave down the bus. Of course, our culture teaches us that losing energy and our physical and mental abilities are natural consequences of aging. Actually, they're very unnatural. If we treat it right, the body is capable of staying healthy into our older years and of dying peacefully as we sleep. Instead, even if we don't have any other harmful lifestyle habits, we are so malnourished that we can be less healthy than someone who eats healthy foods but smokes cigarettes and drinks heavily! Poor nourishment lies at the root of some cancers, diabetes, heart attacks, high cholesterol, hypertension, strokes, and many of the chronic diseases so many of us are suffering and dying from.

Surprisingly, even so-called "superfoods" like broccoli, oatmeal, and soybeans are failing to nourish us adequately. For sure, they're much better for us than highly processed foods; yet research shows that even they have been damaged by "overcivilized practices," the terminology I use to describe the highly industrialized procedures humans use to tinker with nature so they can make more money off the food they grow—overfarming the soil, using synthetic fertilizers, and raising livestock on feed lots. That, to me, is a very sad thing: Even when we think we're taking good care of ourselves, in reality we're not doing nearly enough.

University of California–Berkeley professor of science and environmental journalism Michael Pollan describes our overcivilized processes in his *New York Times* bestseller *The Omnivore's Dilemma: A Natural History of Four Meals.*[3] Pollan describes how produce, grains, poultry, and beef travel from three types of farms—industrial (the mass-production processes that have made traditional farming obsolete), large organic farms, and small family farms—to arrive in your supermarket. (He even bought a calf and tracked what happened to it up to the point that it was slaughtered and made into ground beef.) He compared these processes and the foods they create, contrasting today's processes to how food was raised just a generation or two ago when we cultivated and hunted our own meals. According to Pollan, industrial agricultural practices disrupt the balance of nature, setting in motion a chain reaction whose end product is people whose bodies are weak because they eat poor-quality food. For example, the industrial practice of overfarming the land depletes it of vital nutrients, weakening it and essentially making the soil "sick." Sick soil produces "sick" crops, containing far fewer nutrients than food grown on healthier soil. For over a decade, experts in the wellness industry have cited a statistic that to get the same amount of nutrition out of one cup of spinach grown in 1950, you have to eat between fifteen and twenty cups of spinach today. This dramatic nutritional shortfall exists not just for spinach but for every fruit, vegetable, and grain produced on an industrial farm. Since livestock are fed these grains, they, too, become malnourished. So do humans, who eat not just the impotent crops but the weakened animals raised on them. Sick soil produces sick food, which, in turn, produces sick people.

Eating sick food makes us pile on pounds. Many of us stay hungry and crave certain foods no matter how much we eat. But it's not because the body desperately requires, say, Oreos or

---

[3] Michael Pollan, *The Omnivore's Dilemma: A Natural History of Four Meals* (London: Penguin Press, 2006).

sour-cream-and-onion potato chips; instead, it is seeking missing nutrients. The body craves those foods we've trained it to know it usually obtains certain nutrients from—no matter whether the foods are good for us or not. If we've taught our body that it gets calcium from ice cream, as opposed to yogurt, broccoli, or kale, when it's short on calcium, we will crave cookies 'n' cream rather than greens.

In addition to having a food supply that literally leaves us starved for nourishment, Americans now live in what many experts call a "hostile" food environment—so called because it's easier to find meals that are high in fat, sugar, and salt than it is to get your hands on the fresh, natural, organic foods that Mother Nature intended us to ingest. Most unhealthy foods are also "spiked" with toxins like artificial flavors, colors, preservatives, pesticides, antibiotics, and hormones. Organic foods, in addition to being more difficult to obtain, costs on average 50 percent more than these overcivilized foods, according to *Consumer Reports*. Who can possibly prepare a homemade dinner for the cost of a "99-cent meal deal"? No matter where you get your food—at the fast-food restaurant, the supermarket, or takeout—chances are that if it tastes good and you can get it quickly and inexpensively, it's not very healthy for you.

Thousands of artificial flavors, colors, preservatives, pesticides, hormones, and antibiotics are approved for use in America's food. To know which the body considers noxious, you only need to look at the ingredient label. If you recognize the contents—chicken, vinegar, cayenne pepper, garlic, egg—that ingredient is probably not toxic. But if it contains some chemical or substance you don't recognize, it has the potential to injure you. For fun, check out the ingredient label of some hot dogs, a can of pork and beans, frozen French fries, ketchup, or salad dressing, items containing lots of additives and preservatives. You'll see a couple of familiar ingredients—pork, beans, tomatoes—but the list of chemicals and preservatives is usually longer. You'll see substances like high-fructose corn syrup, monosodium glutamate (MSG), modified food starch, maltodextrine, (artificial) flavor, dextrose, sodium benzoate, xanthan gum, calcium disodium EDTA, caramel color—the

FAQ: Does washing my produce really get rid of pesticides?

A: Washing your fruits and vegetables when you bring them home from the market is always a good idea. In addition to removing dirt and detritus, you're also reducing your risk of catching *E. coli* or another virus from the produce picker's dirty hands (the widely publicized incident where people caught *E. coli* from raw spinach was rare; the vast majority of illness caused by *E. coli* originates with tainted meat). But when it comes to removing pesticides, washing offers mixed results. It may reduce some pesticide residue on the product's surface but it does not wash away substances specifically designed to bind to the surface of the plant, nor does it reduce the amount of pesticide that's been absorbed into the plant itself, according to the EWG. Peeling produce may reduce your exposure, but also many nutrients. So always wash your produce and, following the guidelines on page 51, strategically and as you can afford it, begin to incorporate more organic foods into your diet.

list goes on and on. Eaten individually, none of these ingredients will kill you or make you sick. But the average American eats over two hundred synthetic chemicals daily. On top of that, we're exposed to a hundred non-food toxins. If nature doesn't make it, the body cannot use it effectively. Still, roughly a thousand man-made chemicals are added to America's food supply annually—from artificial "grill flavor" to the preservative I'm sure some scientist somewhere is developing that will keep ice cream from melting in the hot summer sun.

The Dead Zone

Adding insult to injury, in the name of convenience many of the foods we eat have been processed so much that they no longer resemble the product they came from. We eat fruit that has been pressed into portable "roll-ups," processed into frozen dinners in plastic trays, canned so we don't have to shop as often, or knocked off into cheese-foods and other pseudo sauces that make other processed foods taste better. Granted, refined foods are convenient and help us keep up with our fast-paced lives. But when food is boiled and treated with preservatives so it can be canned, it is stripped of nutrients, then enriched so it can be packaged, or is frozen to keep it "fresh" longer, this processing kills the enzymes that help us digest it and phytonutrients (also called phytochemicals), the compounds within the plant that help us protect our health.

Enzymes are the body's workhorses. Found from the top to the bottom of the body, they catalyze all of the chemical reactions that happen inside us—from those that help us blink our eyes to those that allow us to snap our fingers or tap our toes when we're enjoying good music. They also make every organ function. Without them, the body would stop working and we would die. Digestive enzymes, those found in our digestive system, break large molecules of food into smaller particles that can be transported by the blood to the cells. There are four main types of digestive enzymes: *protease* breaks protein down into its building blocks, amino acids; *amylase* dismantles starchy carbs into simple sugars; *lipase* melts fats into essential fatty acids and smaller chains of fatty acids like triglycerides, which many people monitor to prevent heart disease; and *cellulase* dissects fiber. Together, they help the body use food's vitamins and minerals to grow and repair our cells. But as our bodies become more toxic, we become less able to produce these essential enzymes. This problem is compounded when we eat processed or devitalized food that is also short on enzymes. When this happens, the body requires an unnaturally high amount of energy to digest our food, and we get tired after eating. Over time, enzyme shortages weaken our immune system and cause us to fall ill.

Enzymes are so important to our well-being that many nutritional experts label foods whose enzymes have been killed by processing "dead." Natural foods that man hasn't altered are considered to be "alive," even after they've been harvested or slaughtered, because at least some of their enzymes are still living. Those enzymes will diminish and die over the coming days or weeks, depending upon whether they're left out in the sun, on your kitchen counter, or in the refrigerator. Foods whose enzymes are active look, feel, smell, and taste like they're alive; once the enzymes die, the foods look wilted and lifeless.

This fun experiment will help you understand enzymes better: Compare a piece of fresh produce to one that's gotten lost in your refrigerator crisper and has wilted or started to turn color. Now contrast that fresh ingredient to either its frozen or canned counterpart. There's a big difference—the fresher the bean, the more lively it looks and the more snap it has when you bend and break it. The frozen bean's enzymes are dead; however, some of its vitamins and minerals are still living and it's been treated with fewer (if any) preservatives, so it will appear healthier than its canned counterpart. Since it is more alive and less toxic than the canned bean, it will look and taste more fresh. Canned foods not only contain chemical preservatives and no enzymes, but few vitamins and minerals remain in them, and toxins from the can may leach into the food. No wonder canned food looks drab and lifeless and needs artificial colors and flavors added to it! Living foods produce vibrant people. Wilted and tired-looking foods produce wilted and tired people. And dead foods, over time, kill us.

> **FACTOID**
>
> Processing foods kills the naturally occurring enzymes. Dead enzymes equal dead food. You cannot be energetic, vibrant, and lively if you eat dead food.
>
> This is why people experience more energy when they shift from processed to fresh and/or organic foods.

Why do food companies make groceries with items in them that can literally make us sick? Because making food that lasts longer—increasing the amount of "shelf life" it has before it spoils and, consequently, throwing fewer foods away—means companies make a lot more money. But an ancient Chiffon margarine commercial warned, "It's not nice to fool Mother Nature!" As it turns out, the joke is on us—the body doesn't utilize these unnatural nutrients. Of course, that doesn't stop food companies from adding them. Pollan discovered that refining and processing foods allows companies to charge more for the same product. For fun, try to guess what grain comprises the main ingredient of these processed foods?

- Twinkies
- Marshmallows
- Cheetos
- Cheese Whiz
- Sports drinks
- Powdered juice drinks

The answer? Corn. The companies that manufacture these products make more money by charging us higher prices for these processed products than they could ever charge for kernels of corn. I call these and other man-made foods "plastic," since they bear

Pick Your Poison: The 411 on Sugar Substitutes

Among the nation's most common "plastic foods" are the sugar substitutes that sit atop most every table. Every few years, controversy arises over whether these products are healthier than sugar. The answer changes as new research deepens our understanding of the relationship between carbohydrates and insulin.

When we consume overcivilized, refined sugars like white sugar and high-fructose corn syrup, glucose (the form of sugar our body uses for energy) surges into our bloodstream. The pancreas then sprints into action as it tries to release the hormone insulin into the bloodstream fast enough for the brain and body to use the glucose for energy. When we eat natural, complex sweeteners like honey, maple syrup, and molasses, glucose still enters our bloodstream but at a much slower pace. This allows the pancreas to release insulin more comfortably. Because it can work at a more reasonable pace, the organ doesn't wear itself out sprinting and hitting the brakes over and over again—or, more accurately, given how much refined sugar most of us eat—by sprinting, then sprinting again and again. All of that revving up exhausts the pancreas, often causing diabetes. Any excess sugar it doesn't move quickly enough to use gets converted to fat. And because the sugar is converted to energy so quickly, it leaves us craving more food soon after.

Many people use artificial sweeteners to stay thin and avoid the cycle of sugar highs and lows. But as many problems as white sugar causes, I believe it is healthier than sugar substitutes, which include aspartame, acesulfame, neutame, sucralose, and alitame—more commonly known as Nutrasweet and Equal (blue packages), Splenda (yellow package), and Sweet'N Low and saccharin (pink packages). However, neither white sugar nor the synthetic sugar substitutes are as healthy as stevia, a sweetening herb from South America that is available in green packets in select locations. Here's the skinny on the artificial sweeteners many people take to avoid getting fat.

Aspartame

Sold as Nutrasweet and Equal, aspartame produces toxins that can harm the brain and mental functions. It also blocks serotonin production, interfering with users' ability to experience pleasure and contributing to depression in many people. Aspartame also robs the body of chromium, a valuable mineral that helps control blood sugar. And because it's unnatural and therefore doesn't nourish us, aspartame starves our cells of nutrients, causing cravings and weight gain.

Saccharin

The oldest of the artificial sugars, saccharin, used in Sweet'N Low, is derived from a plant imported from China. The FDA describes it as a complex natural sugar, so I find it strange that the FDA used to require it to sport this warning label: "Use of this product may be hazardous to your health. This product contains saccharin, which has been determined to cause cancer in laboratory animals." For some reason, the FDA has recently changed its tune, refuting the cancer claim and allowing the warning label to be removed.

Stevia

If you're looking for a sugar substitute, I suggest using stevia. You don't need much of it—according to studies, it's thirty times sweeter than sugar. Yet it does not raise blood sugar levels, causing the pancreas to sprint to produce insulin, or cause rapid-onset cravings the way simple sugars do. A study published in the *Journal of Ethno-Pharmacology* found that stevia dilates the blood vessels and helps to prevent high blood pressure. It helps to regulate the digestive system, encourages the growth of friendly bacteria, and helps us detoxify the body and excrete more urine naturally.

Sucralose

Sucralose contains chlorine, a toxin research shows causes cancer. A little bit of chlorine stays in the body with each packet of Splenda we use. Sucralose also shrinks the thymus gland and enlarges the liver and kidney in rodents. In humans, scientists know that it causes our cells to mutate slowly, eventually causing cancer. Some people experience more immediate side effects, including dizziness, numbness, panic-like agitation, and intestinal cramping.

no resemblance to the products they're made from. These days, the vast majority of Americans are living on plastic foods.

Gluttons for Punishment?

Not only do Americans eat harmful food, we eat way too much of it. In fact, we eat so much food that Pollan believes we have a "national eating disorder." I agree. Only one generation ago, people ate three square meals a day and perhaps a snack. They drank milk, water, and maybe some orange juice for breakfast or an occasional soda for a treat. Folks socialized and had fun without food's being involved. Today, eating is the focus of almost everything. There's a good chance we'll be chowing down whether we're exercising (sports drinks, flavored waters, energy bars), at our child's basketball game (soda, hot dogs, candy), socializing (chips, beer, soda, ice cream), dating (dinner dates), watching TV (chips, beer, soda, hot wings, pizza), meeting clients (power lunches, drinks, business dinners), or picking up the kids from soccer practice (fast food). Turn on the TV and what do you see? Food, food, food! And let's not forget beverages. The average American teenager drinks twenty-two ounces of soft drinks and fruit drinks (13 percent of their calories) each day compared to just nine ounces of milk, according to *Liquid Candy: How Soft Drinks Are Harming Americans' Health*, a report published by consumer watchdogs Center for Science in the Public Interest (CSPI).[4] Soda pop has bumped milk off the top of the list of beverages young people drink most. Americans literally eat and drink all day long—and we don't see anything wrong with it.

How did an entire society's eating habits change so quickly? According to one of the nation's leading nutritionists, Marion Nestle, PhD, MPH, professor and former chair of the department of nutrition, food studies, and public health at New York University, Americans are experiencing the flip side of what she calls the "paradox of plenty." During most of human history, the food supply has been erratic. Our bodies literally adapted to survive in either "feast or famine," primarily famine since food has usually not been plentiful. But we've advanced so quickly technologically that American industry now produces an overabundance of food, particularly corn and soybeans. In fact, if you add up the number of calories each person living in America needs to maintain a healthy weight and compare that to the number of calories food companies produce, you'd find there's twice as much food available as we need to be healthy. Not surprisingly, food producers want to sell as much of this food as profitably as they can. Their strategies range from inventing innovative (read: overcivilized) products and making them look sumptuous in television ads to lobbying government officials to buying out experts to advertising to children, who don't know that they're being manipulated. It does not matter to them if selling more food occurs at the expense of public

---

[4] Michael F. Jacobson; *Liquid Candy: How Soft Drinks Are Harming Americans' Health* (Washington, DC: CSPI, 2005).

health, Dr. Nestle writes in her book *Food Politics: How the Food Industry Influences Nutrition and Health*. "The leading [health] conditions related to diet—coronary heart disease, cancers at certain sites, diabetes, stroke, and liver cirrhosis, for example—could be reduced in prevalence or delayed until later in life if people ate less of the dietary components that increase disease risk. Advice to eat less, however, runs counter to the interest of food producers."[5]

In an interview on Amazon.com's streaming video show *Amazon Fishbowl*, Pollan charges that Americans are "deliberately confused by an industry that spends $36 billion a year on marketing messages precisely to persuade us to eat more, and eat at different times, eat in the car, eat in front of television, and eat highly processed foods, because that's where the money is." Dr. Nestle says the food industry intentionally keeps us confused about whether foods like chocolate, coffee, and eggs are good or bad for us and whether food labels like "low fat," "low calorie" and "natural" really mean as much as they imply. Though I am not an expert on food industry economics, recently I witnessed an example of food-marketing hype firsthand. I saw packages of carrots that were labeled low fat. A low-fat label on a carrot? What nonsense! Of course they're low fat—they're carrots!

Food manufacturers do so much marketing—and very effectively—that they have changed the meaning of food from something we use to nourish ourselves, which is how we thought of it only one generation ago, to something we consume whenever we want to celebrate something, nourish, reward, comfort, or rev ourselves up. No wonder so many of us now live to eat rather than eat to live.

Where does the government stand on all of this? Some experts charge that the FDA experiences a conflict of interest inherent in its mission statement: that it must choose between promoting foods American farmers grow and directing consumers not to eat too much. "No government agency has the funds to promote dietary recommendations in competition with food advertising,"

---

[5] Marion Nestle, *Food Politics: How the Food Industry Influences Nutrition and Health* (Berkeley: University of California Press, 2002).

Dr. Nestle writes. As a result, she claims, "The major sources of nutrition advice for most people are the media and the public relations efforts of the food industry itself." In his 2004 testimony before Congress in hearings to evaluate the government's role in curbing obesity, Bruce Silverglade, legal affairs director for CSPI, explained to congressional panel members that food company marketing budgets alone dwarf those of the government's healthy-eating campaign—$7 *billion* to $4 to $5 million. It's no surprise, then, that the message that Americans should eat less doesn't get emphasized.

How Being Too Toxic Makes You Fat

If you look under a microscope at somebody's blood right after they've eaten, you can see how the food they've eaten is affecting their body. During my studies, we used to do an experiment where we would ask people to eat a typical American convenience meal—say, fast food or pizza—then we'd draw their blood and examine it. If their diet was at all healthy, when we'd look at their blood cells before they ate, we'd see circular cells with space between them. But after a fast-food meal, the space between the blood cells was gone. Instead, they would be crowded next to and stacked on top of one another. We would show these "before and after" pictures to the volunteers. They'd be shocked to witness in their blood cells proof of why they felt sluggish and tired. Next, we'd ask them to consume five to ten digestive enzymes, whose job it is to eat up all the crud, allowing cells to swim in oxygenated blood. In less than an hour, the person would feel better and become more energetic. When we looked at their cells under the microscope, we could see that the cells were less crowded and able to breathe.

On a molecular level, when toxins enter the body in our food, the body tries to digest them. Once it realizes it's dealing with something unnatural, it mobilizes more and more enzymes as it tries (unsuccessfully) to break down the synthetic ingredients. When we feel ourselves becoming tired, bloated, gassy; experiencing heartburn, GERD (gastroesophageal reflux disease), or an upset stomach; getting diarrhea; or even becoming constipated, this is often the reason why. It's also the reason 20 percent of Americans have digestive problems, and digestive aids like Tums, Milk of Magnesia, Pepcid, Prilosec, Zantac, Gas-X, and Imodium AD are among the best-selling over-the-counter and prescription medications. Eventually, the body realizes these substances are indigestible (hmm . . . that's awfully similar to the word *indigestion*). At that point, it moves them out of the stomach to the colon, one of the body's major trash cans. But even the colon doesn't know what to do with them. After sitting there for a while—constipating us, causing gas, body odor, and other problems as it tries to figure out what to do—they migrate into the lymphatic system, the body's drainage network. When the lymph system doesn't know how to deal with them, it dumps these toxins into our fat cells, whose primary job is to cushion and insulate our organs, but whose side gig is to store trash.

Over the course of our lifetime, as more toxins are shoved into our fat cells—on top of the fat—the cells get crowded and congested. When they get congested, we feel congested. We also develop cellulite, which is merely garbage stored in our fat cells that isn't supposed to be there. As our fat cells are stuffed fuller and fuller, we bloat, we get heavier, our clothes get tight. Over time, our cells become crowded so closely together that they can't get enough oxygen. In an effort to find someplace to put the junk we pile into it, our body creates more fat cells. They, too, get crammed full of crap until they can't take it anymore. They begin to wither, become misshapen and their growth becomes retarded. Eventually, they literally suffocate. Making matters worse, these overcivilized foods turn the colon, kidneys, and liver—organs whose job it is to filter harmful items out of the bloodstream and remove them from the body—into toxic cesspools. Over time, they become overloaded and unable to function, literally leaving us sick and tired. We are able to feel that something's not right with us, but because the problem exists at a microscopic level, only the most knowledgeable people are aware of exactly what's going on. The rest of us wonder why we feel symptoms like fatigue, sluggishness, foggy thinking, confusion, headaches, allergies, and body aches. This toxicity manifests itself in more noticeable ways, including symptoms like wrinkles, age spots, skin that is overly dry or oily, acne, allergies, and body odor.

By the time we're experiencing these types of signs, we're usually quite overweight. Before long, we'll experience signs of *chemical onslaught* or *toxic overload*. Our blood pressure starts to creep up; our cholesterol rises; our head, joints, and body ache. These are signs society teaches us are natural consequences of aging, but they have nothing to do with our age. They're actually telltale proof that we're toxic. (A body that is properly nourished, well cared for, and protected from toxins of all types will function well until we're in our nineties, and the person will die quietly in their sleep.) At this point, we usually go to the doctor. But "American physicians are not trained to look for the unavoidably ubiquitous environmental causes of disease. Nor are they trained in how to get them out of the body to reverse disease," Dr. Rogers writes. Instead, they prescribe medication. The medication alleviates the symptoms that were bothering us, but it gives us "side effects," a euphemism for the toxic consequences of the drugs. We then return to our doctor because we have these new symptoms. *Many people's bodies become so overloaded with toxins that it is physically impossible for them to lose weight by using traditional dieting methods.* Once people reach this point, no matter what they do, how diligent they are, what kind of diet they try, or how strictly they stick with it, there is no traditional dieting approach that will help shed excess pounds. Toxins have actually mucked up their biochemistry. *Being fat is not their fault.*

Consider the case of trans fats, often contained in buttery spreads, fast foods, baked goods, chips, dips, and packaged and frozen foods. One reason scientists now warn us away from these fats is their toxicity. To allow vegetable oils to last longer before they spoil and to make them solid at room temperature (think: many margarines and shortening), manufacturers began to tinker with their molecular structure, adding hydrogen to the oils, a process called hydrogenation. Hydrogenation actually alters the shape of the oil molecules, making trans fats worse for you than saturated (animal) fats such as butter. And like the "roach motels" that claim that roaches can check in but they can't check out, hydrogenated oils can enter your cells but your cell can't figure out how to expel them. They gunk up the cells' inner workings, increasing low-density lipoprotein (LDL—bad) cholesterol, which increases your heart attack risk, while lowering high-density lipoprotein (HDL—good) cholesterol, which protects against it. It's no surprise, then, that they interfere with our ability to lose weight, cause us to store weight in our midsection, and age more quickly. Trans fats are so dangerous that the FDA now requires them to be listed on food ingredient labels. Unfortunately, this is not the case in restaurants, where it's hard to know how your food is being prepared—unless you live in New York City or a short list of other communities that have banned trans fats altogether.

In addition to this troublesome toxin, many of us have problems with our metabolic system, including the common issues described below:

Insulin Resistance/Metabolic Resistance/Syndrome X

With a name as cryptic as syndrome X, you'd think that insulin resistance was a mysterious disease unique to a James Bond movie. In reality, this physical response to excess sugar in the bloodstream is becoming an increasingly common precursor to diseases like diabetes, high blood pressure, high cholesterol, obesity, and kidney disease. After we eat, the body breaks our food down into glucose and other substances, which the cells use for energy. Before the cells can actually use the glucose, however, it has to be transported inside them. That's where insulin comes in. The pancreas secretes insulin, the hormone that transports glucose to the cells, then unlocks the doors or *receptor sites* so the glucose can get inside. Sometimes these receptors malfunction and the doors to the cells won't open. When this happens, too much glucose and insulin remain in the bloodstream. The pancreas senses that it isn't needed so it kicks back into low gear, over time becoming lazy. In the meantime, the blood sugar that's locked out of the cells continues to circulate around the body looking for places to store itself as fat. As this happens, the affected person experiences a low energy level.

Hormone Imbalance

From insulin to testosterone, the body is brimming with hormones, chemical messengers that ferry information between cells. For many reasons—not infrequently, interference from toxins—our hormones can get out of balance. When they do, they alter our body function as well as our metabolic rate. Consider what happens when the metabolism-controlling thyroid hormone thyroxin drops too low: hypothyroidism develops, slowing the metabolism and causing weight gain. People also develop dry skin and dry and brittle hair and nails that break easily. Doctors usually prescribe a thyroid hormone, but it can affect the menstrual cycle, causing a new set of woes. Conversely, when thyroxin levels rise too high, we tend to lose weight.

Parasites

Most intestinal parasites are foreign to the body but live in the intestines, where they feed off of the body, to its detriment. Some sources claim that 85 percent of North Americans have one or more of these pests, which include leaches to hookworms to tapeworms and range in size from being microscopic up to eight feet long. According to data from the United Nations, over 1.5 billion people worldwide have roundworms. A chronic case of parasites interferes with the body's metabolism. They prevent it from absorbing nutrients and trigger it to produce too much yeast, making our body overly acidic and our organs sluggish, compromising the immune system and creating toxins. Parasites have caused many of my clients' digestive and colon problems. Frankly, I believe they are far more common than the medical community is willing or able to address.

Prescription Drugs

From antihistamines for allergies to beta blockers for blood pressure, to diabetes and antidepressant meds, to hormones like birth control pills and hormone replacement therapy (HRT), medications can alter your metabolism, making it difficult, if not impossible, to lose weight. Medicine introduces chemicals into your bloodstream the body didn't intend to be there. In addition to causing side effects that may be worse than the disorder, these chemicals slow the metabolism and cause people to pick up pounds.

For example, many women have hormone problems, most often a condition called *estrogen dominance*, where there is more estrogen in the body than progesterone. Excess estrogen not only causes women to retain fluid and become irritable, it causes the blood sugar to become imbalanced, causing many women to crave sugar or carbohydrates, which, in turn, cause the body to create fat. Ugh! No wonder women know that if they go on the Pill, HRT, or other hormones, they are likely to get heavy. If a woman has too much estrogen in her system, she tends to retain fluid, gain weight, bloat, and become irritable.

When the antidepressant medications Prozac, Zoloft, Paxil, and Celexa were brought to the market, the manufacturers originally claimed they would cause weight loss. Nonsense! Many people who take antidepressants find that they pick up pounds. Sometimes it's because the drugs increase their appetite; in other cases, it slows their metabolism. Even over-the-counter sleeping pills cause water retention.

When my patients learn that the meds they thought were helping them are causing them to gain weight, they inevitably want to stop taking their pills. But this, too, can be dangerous. I always recommend that my clients consult with their doctor before discontinuing any medication. That said, there are many natural approaches to treating common health conditions. For instance, many people find that essential fatty acids relieve their depression, and garlic capsules are an age-old and effective approach to decreasing blood pressure. For more information about treating medical problems with natural remedies, I suggest *Natural Cures* by Kevin Trudeau[6] or the classic *Prescription for Nutritional Healing* by Phyllis and James Balch.[7] It is important to keep your physician in the loop. For instance, natural approaches like herbs can interact with other medicines, causing unwanted reactions.

Sluggish Metabolism

When the body doesn't get enough oxygen, it becomes sluggish and the metabolism slows, making it harder to lose weight. This can occur among smokers, people who have asthma and are unable to breathe deeply, and those who don't exercise or are chronically ill and unable to move much.

Smoking

Many people keep smoking just to keep from gaining weight. Nicotine artificially elevates the heart rate, stimulates feel-good areas of our brain by elevating our dopamine pathways, increases the metabolism, suppresses the appetite, and causes the liver to release glycogen, which is basically stored glucose (sugar). As it enters into the bloodstream, glycogen raises the blood sugar slightly, making you feel less hungry.

And let's not ignore the reality that many people become accustomed to putting something in their mouth. When the person stops smoking and nicotine is no longer in their system, the metabolism slows to its normal level and blood-sugar levels fall, making them feel hungrier. Even if they keep eating at their normal rate, they will, of course, gain weight. And as their dopamine pathways return to normal levels, they may overeat, pick fights, or create outrageous fears in an attempt to induce the body's fight-or-flight pathways to give them the dopamine fix they're used to. When people quit smoking, they should expect to be hungry and

---

[6] Kevin Trudeau, *Natural Cures "They" Don't Want You to Know About* (New York: Alliance Publishing, 2005).

[7] Phyllis and James Balch, *Prescription for Nutritional Healing*, 4th ed. (New York: Avery, 2006).

irritable for 30 days. What's the best medicine? Exercise. It stimulates a dopamine rush and metabolism!

Yeast Overgrowth

Everyone's body contains at least a little yeast, which is a type of fungus. There are three major causes of disease, fungus being one of them (viruses and bacteria are the other two, with parasites in hot pursuit). Excess yeast causes a variety of symptoms, depending on the person. Common signs include vaginal yeast infections among women, rashes that can develop under large breasts, male jock itch, and athlete's foot. When there is so much yeast in the body that it overwhelms the entire system, it is called *Candida*, which places a significant strain on the immune system. The allopathic medical community acknowledges that *Candida* exists, but traditional practitioners mistakenly believe that you have to be half dead to have it. They're wrong. Between the time people experience a yeast infection or jock itch and the time it becomes systemic, they experience many symptoms of the fungus's spread, including extreme fatigue, serious brain fog, weight gain or loss, craving carbohydrates and sweets, and thrush in their mouth, which is common among people with AIDS. When a person who has *Candida* is also sensitive to mold, the combination can suppress the metabolism, depleting the body of vital energy. When this happens, the body gains weight.

The Three Levels of Food

Fortunately, a lot of people are waking up to the presence of toxins in their lives. Folks used to give me funny looks when I'd talk to them about poisons in our food and bodies. Now they tell me, "I know I'm toxic! I need to eat more organic foods." According to the Organic Trade Association, organic food sales have consistently increased by between 15 percent and 21 percent annually since 1997. More organic foods are becoming available in mainstream grocery and food stores. In fact, the two largest health-food chains, Whole Foods and Wild Oats, now account for less than

The Three Levels of Food

Level 1: Overcivilized Food

What it is: The highly processed and refined food often found in a supermarket's middle aisles that's been making so many Americans fat and sick.

Examples: There are different types of overcivilized food. Of the different varieties, frozen foods are best for you; fast foods and prepared foods are worse; and canned, boxed, and instant varieties are the least healthy for you. The prepared foods you buy in the supermarket are typically frozen foods that have been put in the microwave. They come loaded with extra salt, sugar, and chemicals.

What's wrong with it: High in sugar, salt, preservatives, unhealthy fats, antibiotics, and pesticides, and low in fiber, nutrients, and enzymes.

What it does to you: Weakens your immune system, leaving you vulnerable to colds, viruses, and chronic diseases, like diabetes and hypertension.

How it makes you feel: Tired, confused, heavy.

Level 2: Fresh and Organic Food

What it is: Whole foods eaten in the form in which nature made them, ideally without chemical preservatives, hormones, pesticides, and antibiotics.

Examples: There are several levels of organic foods. Fresh organic fruits, vegetables, whole grains, and meats are best for you, followed by fresh nonorganic foods. Frozen fruits and vegetables retain many vitamins and often don't contain as many preservatives as packaged and canned foods, but they lack vital enzymes needed for the body to digest them properly. Frozen dinners and canned, boxed, and instant foods are the least of the healthy organic options because they often contain sugar, salt, preservatives, and unhealthy fats.

What's wrong with it: Fresh organic and nonorganic foods are far less toxic than overcivilized food, though they are still exposed to our polluted water and air, and nonorganic foods are treated with chemicals as they are grown. In general, the more processed an organic or nonorganic food is, the less of a health benefit it offers. However, processed organic foods are usually healthier for you than processed nonorganic or overcivilized foods.

What it does to you: Organic foods support good health and help you maintain a healthy weight or lose weight, as well as detoxify. Try to eat organic or fresh foods as often as possible.

How it makes you feel: Strong, clear-headed, energetic.

Level 3: High-Density Nutritional Supplements

What it is: When we use it as nature intended, food can not only nourish us and keep us healthy, it can help us heal far better than any prescription medication. When we consume high-density nutritional supplements, we're using food as medicine.

Examples: Green powder, antioxidant drinks, protein powder, cleansing herbs, high-powered phytonutrients (plant compounds thought to have health-promoting qualities), vitamins, minerals, enzymes, amino acids, essential fatty acids, and so on.

What's wrong with it: May be more expensive than traditional medicine, though definitely less expensive than getting sick.

What it does to you: Strengthens the immune system, balances hormones, protects against degenerative diseases, promotes weight loss, supports detoxification.

How it makes you feel: Strong, clear-headed, more energetic than eating organic foods alone.

half of organic food sales, as supermarkets, mass merchandisers, and even Wal-Mart have gotten in on the act.

This shift to organic is proof that increasing numbers of people want to eat higher up on the food chain, moving up what I call the three levels of food: from overcivilized processed and refined foods back to the civilized, wholesome, and healthy foods our parents and grandparents ate. By making this shift, we get back to nature, not only to provide the body with more of the nutrition it needs to function healthily but also to keep ourselves disease free by supporting it in regenerating itself and purging poisons. As we make this shift, we release ourselves from the physical, mental, and spiritual dis-ease we feel when we're uncomfortable in our own bodies and free ourselves from being imprisoned by a lifetime of unsuccessful dieting.

How Can I Afford to Eat Organic?

Who wouldn't want to eat foods with fewer pesticides, hormones, and antibiotics in them—if only they could afford them, my clients tell me. "You have to be rich to eat organic," they complain. Organic foods are definitely more costly than conventional items. They are more expensive to grow and are not subsidized by the government as conventional foods are. As a result, according to *Consumer Reports* (CR), you'll pay 50 percent more, on average, for organic items.

Fortunately, there are ways to reduce your exposure to food toxins without turning your pockets inside out. The following guidelines, developed by CR, can help you identify when buying organic is smart and when to save your coins.

Buy organic as often as possible: Apples, carrots, celery, cherries, imported grapes, nectarines, peaches, pears, potatoes, red raspberries, spinach, strawberries; meat, poultry, eggs, dairy products; baby food.

Buy organic if you can afford it: Asparagus, avocados, bananas, broccoli, cauliflower, kiwi, mangos, onions, papaya, pineapples, peas (sweet); breads, oils, potato chips, pasta, cereals, and other packaged foods like frozen and canned fruits and vegetables.

Don't bother buying organic: Seafood; cosmetics.

2

DETOXING VS. DIETING

What's the Difference?

When I was growing up, my siblings and I would spend summers with my grandmother down in Greenville, North Carolina. Grandma has always been a very healthy woman, in every sense of the word—spiritually, mentally, and physically. She prays often, reads her Bible daily, and goes to church religiously. A model of Christian temperance, in my entire life I've never seen her smoke a cigarette, drink an alcoholic beverage, ride in the car without her seat belt, or anything else unhealthy or unsafe. In fact, I've never even seen her eat junk food!

During my childhood, Grandma would go outside each morning and pick tomatoes, string beans, greens, cabbage, and other vegetables from her garden. Then she'd spend the day doing what so many Southern women of her generation did—cook, cook, cook! She'd prepare big pots of collard greens, turnips, and black-eyed peas, as well as corn bread and chicken. Then she'd make us big plates of food, saying, "Kids have to grow, so you eat up." She also dished out huge servings for her husband, Granddaddy Bruce, who ate so much food we children thought it was funny. After he ate, Granddaddy would kick back in his easy chair, put up his feet, fall asleep, and start snoring.

But Grandma never ate as much food as she made. She'd

say, "Grandma can't eat that much food—I'll get tired and fall asleep!"

In my entire life I've never seen Grandma eat a big meal. She was what you would call a "grazer." She'd dish herself out a little plate of collard greens and eat them. In a few hours she would nibble on some okra and string beans. After a short time she might have some cornbread and a little piece of meat. Later, she'd enjoy a potato. Grandma nibbled all day long, but she was never overweight. She ate just enough food to satisfy her hunger—nothing more, nothing less.

This type of mindfulness and self-awareness extended to her basic lifestyle habits. When it was time for us to go somewhere, we kids would always be in a rush.

"Come on, Grandma. Let's go!" we would tell her.

But Grandma had a very calm nature. She never let anybody rush her. "You all go on," she'd say. "Grandma's going to sit right here and tend to her business."

"Business" meant that she would not leave the house unless she had eaten, had a bowel movement, and was presentably dressed. I remember sitting and waiting on many occasions until she had finished "doing her business" in the bathroom. When she was done, she'd say, "Let's go! Now I'm ready to do whatever you want." And she would.

Like many women of her era, Grandma relied on the old ways of healing. Because our family didn't have a lot of money, there was no such thing as going to the doctor. We relied on traditional methods to keep us from getting sick. If I started getting the sniffles or an upset stomach, Grandma would say, "Come here, gal, and take this cod liver oil." It was either that or castor oil—one would give me diarrhea, the other would make me throw up. Either way, she'd flush the "bug" out. On the rare occasions when I did come down with something, she would slather me with Vicks, top me off with onions and garlic, and wrap me in wet hot towels, then a plastic bag to help me sweat the virus out. At the time, of course, I thought it was the most horrible thing, but now that I think back on it, I realize that it worked: I'd get the chills, start sweating, and immediately get better.

Only once in my life have I known Grandma to feel under the weather. I was in my mid-twenties when it happened. For some reason, family members had reached the conclusion that Grandma had high blood pressure. Being the family's only nurse, everyone wanted me to take care of her. I figured I'd take her to the doctor. She didn't want to go.

"You've gotta go get some medicine, Grandma," I told her. Of course, this was back in the days when I still believed that the best way to treat a health problem was with prescription medication.

"I don't have high blood pressure," she told me. Grandma was stubborn; she insisted her blood pressure was normal. But after I begged and begged and begged her, she finally gave in and agreed to go to the doctor.

When we got to the doctor, we learned that Grandma's blood pressure was sky high. The doctor handed Grandma a prescription for antihypertensive medication. She refused to take it.

"There's nothing wrong with my blood pressure," she insisted. The fact that she wouldn't take the medicine worried me. With a reading that high, I was afraid she'd have a stroke. So when we got home, I took her blood pressure again. To my surprise the reading was very low: 96 over 70. I called the doctor and told him.

"That's impossible!" he told me. "You have to bring her back in. There's something wrong with your machine."

Grandma was adamant: "I'm not going back to the doctor." But we children and grandchildren kept insisting. Eventually, she relented and let me take her back in. Once again, her blood pressure reading was sky high! I took her back home and took her reading again. Her blood pressure had dropped to a healthy level. "I don't have high blood pressure."

Finally, it occurred to me that maybe there was a reason her blood pressure was high every time she went to the doctor: fear was driving her blood pressure up. It's called "white-coat" hypertension—literally, fear of the doctor or medical settings! I would never recommend that anyone with high blood pressure refuse to take their medication; yet I'm very glad my grandmother listened to her instincts. She didn't need an antihypertensive.

Had she taken the medication, it undoubtedly would have made her sick or possibly killed her.

The experience taught me that it's possible to be so in tune with yourself that you know whether something is wrong with you better than any doctor does, better than any instrument or machine. Unfortunately, few of us live that way anymore. Few of us are that self-aware.

Today, I understand that Grandma is a paradigm of good health—eating fresh foods, using the bathroom regularly, listening to her body, tending to her spirit, moving to her own rhythm, detoxifying herself regularly, and healing herself with natural methods. She has not only outlived her spouse, who died at a young age, she's survived the loss of most of her friends and some of her children. Yet she has never needed medication. In addition to giving me unconditional love and a lifetime of amazing memories, I realize that she has given me a very precious gift: she role-modeled the kinds of choices you make when you take good care of yourself. As of the writing of this book, she's closing in on a hundred years old.

The Gift of Our Inner Wisdom

Many things that Grandma knew by listening to her own mind, body, and spirit, researchers now know scientifically. For instance, we've learned that the body has inner wisdom, that our spirit is real, and that prayer can heal. Research has demonstrated the healthful benefits of eating fresh foods and a balanced diet. We now understand that it is important to have regular bowel movements and that grazing is healthier than consuming big meals. We've also learned that systematic undereating is an antiaging technique. A growing body of research shows that in a variety of animal species, those who are optimally nourished, yet eat about 30 percent fewer calories than average, live longer and healthier lives. Calorie restriction has not been studied extensively on humans because we live such long lives; however, studies published in such reputable journals as the *Journal of the American*

Medical Association and *New England Journal of Medicine* suggest that people who eat less live longer.

Most of us have drifted away from this and other natural wisdom common among our elders and ancestors. In its place we have embraced a culture that encourages us not to care for our bodies and a lifestyle that depletes our energy. In my practice I'm seeing an increasing number of people who want to get back to a simpler, cleaner way of life. They want to go back to nature, back to their roots. I think that approach is smart. Losing weight and keeping it off and preventing and healing from chronic diseases requires that we adopt a more natural way of life.

Human life is a miracle, yet I don't believe it's an accident. Accidents are, by nature, disorganized; human existence requires and contains far more order than any doctor or scientist can comprehend. Many researchers, who by nature and discipline are very objective, are reaching the conclusion that the level of organization is so profound that God has to exist. I believe that we are made for a purpose and are the end result of a process that is far more complex than we will ever understand. We are an essential part of nature. Our ancestors and many indigenous ethnic groups today "got" this and treated the natural world with respect. Western culture discourages us from understanding our vital yet delicate relationship with nature and we are suffering for it. If we understood how closely linked we are, we would not pollute, destroy, or disrespect the Earth. For when we endanger the health of the planet, we endanger ourselves. Consider this example illustrating our basic interconnectedness: When plants and trees lose their leaves, they release oxygen into the atmosphere. To state it simply, we humans breathe that oxygen into our lungs. From there it flows into our bloodstream and out to our cells. The cells use oxygen to power our muscles; without it, they stop working. As the body uses oxygen, it converts it to carbon dioxide, which the bloodstream carries back to the lungs, which emit it into the air when we exhale. Plants and trees breathe this carbon dioxide in and use it to conduct photosynthesis, the most important biochemical reaction on the planet: the process by which plants convert sunlight into energy, which we, in turn, obtain from our food. But if we keep cutting down trees, which create oxygen, and burning fossil fuels, like coal, oil, and natural gas, which release unnatural amounts of carbon dioxide into our environment, how will our species survive?

Just as our society dissuades us from understanding nature, it discourages us from understanding our bodies. Do you ever wonder what makes your heart beat? Why you blink your eyes? How your fingernails grow? Why you have body hair? Each of these functions is important. Consider this: every physical, mental, and emotional feature you display exists for a specific reason. The body, which we tend to think of either in its entirety or in terms of body parts—nice hands, a pretty face, too much cellulite, aching knees—is actually a collection of trillions of individual cells designed to act in perfect harmony and organization. Each of those trillions of cells has its own internal engine that powers it and brain that tells it what to do. Each cell breathes the oxygen and consumes the nutrients our blood carries around our bodies. Instead of opening their mouths, they open their membranes to permit vital elements and nutrients to enter them. When they're through eating, they eliminate waste.

Each of these trillion cells has its unique purpose and cooperates with other cells to carry out some essential function. For example, one set of cells forms our skeleton, a framework of connections holding approximately two hundred bones together and protecting our vital organs and soft tissues, like the heart, stomach, and reproductive system. Other cells make up the body's defense team, whose job it is to protect us from injury. For example, our lymph nodes filter out invading viruses, bacteria, and foreign substances. Among the spleen's many functions is purifying our blood of toxins. The liver transports blood from the spleen, stomach, pancreas, and intestine and cleans any invaders—for instance, bacteria, viruses, fungi, foreign chemicals, and other toxins—out of it before sending it into the sensitive circulatory system.

While performing their specific functions, our cells are constantly communicating with each other. The *central nervous sys-*

tem (CNS) governs, regulates, and directs this communication; oversees the cells that manage our mental activity, including those that help us think, learn, and remember; and supervises cells engaged in specific activities that take place in a short period of time, like blinking our eyes or running away from a dog. The *endocrine system*, which controls hormones—for example, testosterone for male reproduction; estrogen for female reproduction; and insulin, which is responsible for sugar metabolism—manages those cells engaged in longer-term processes, like metabolizing food and growing. The latest advances in human technology can't hold a candle to the intricate ways our cells communicate. If the spleen becomes injured and is unable to purify our blood, the CNS sends a message to the liver to take over its job. The liver also steps up if our kidneys become weak. However, I'm not sure if the cells take on this extra work willingly or if they have a bad attitude because the other organ is not pulling its weight.

Each cell has a natural life cycle whose duration depends on the role it plays. The lifespan of a skin cell is shorter than that of a bone cell. Red blood cells, for example, live for 120 days, while a certain type of nerve cell hangs around for up to 100 years. At its appointed time, each cell will birth a baby cell that is an exact duplicate of itself. The health of the baby cell depends on the well-being of its parent. A variety of factors can affect cell wellness, which can range from healthy to sick to someplace in between. Cells become ill when they don't get enough oxygen; for example, the person may have anemia, which may be caused by a shortage of red blood cells that transport oxygen around the body; they don't eat enough nutrients; they are exposed to extreme cold or heat; they experience trauma, such as electric shock or radiation treatment, which destroy cells; or they are exposed to toxins. Once damaged, our cells begin to feel "off," and may malfunction, shrink, wither, and even die before their time. While our cells never stop working, they may slow down because they are out of balance or their organization is threatened. The way our cells feel affects how our body feels. If our cells are not working right or are out of balance, we sense it.

Under normal conditions and when our cells are healthy, if

they get injured or out of alignment, they automatically heal or balance themselves. Perfect health is the body's natural condition, the state that it innately strives to achieve. Although we rarely think of the body as wanting to be well, we all have personal experiences that prove it. Who does not have childhood memories of, say, falling off their bicycle and skinning their knee? We bled, the body's way of cleansing the wound, and a loved one wiped it with an antiseptic solution and bandaged it. A few days later when we removed the dressing we discovered that our body had created a scab and new skin. Our body heals us even if we fall again, scraping off the scab. Even if we pick off that scab intentionally, the skin beneath will keep on healing time and time again. Though the idea of getting cancer scares most people to death, we successfully fight off cancerous cells every day of our life. If ultimately they overrun us, it's only after decades during which our self-healing mechanisms effectively kept them in check. Unless we're ill, all through our life our paper cuts, hangnails, scratches, cold sores, bone breaks, and bruises repair themselves.

But while we know from personal experience that the body has the ability to self-heal, we live in a culture whose indigenous healing arts have been destroyed, that teaches that the body can't be trusted and that it's the doctor or medicine that heals us. It's no wonder we forget! No matter what health care professionals or pharmaceutical companies imply, medicines do not and cannot make us better. Medicine may alleviate symptoms, but it's our body that heals us. The body's repair department is on call 24 hours a day, 365 days yearly. It heals us without our conscious effort or knowledge because being healthy is our nature. Only some of the functions the nervous system coordinates are activities that our mind has power over. Other activities happen whether we want them to or not. No matter how hard we may try, the average person cannot, for instance, change their skin, hair, or eye color (naturally); will themselves to grow taller; change their body type; or get rid of their naturally skinny calves or their propensity to have a prominent posterior. (I say the "average person" because some people have trained themselves to exercise mind power over physical matter, to self-heal or accomplish amazing feats like walking on hot coals.) It is also impossible to stop the body from attempting to heal.

No matter how well or poorly we treat it, the body always attempts to create a state of balance, called *equilibrium* or *homeostasis*. It doesn't matter how off center we are—whether we stay so busy at work that we consistently skip lunch, whether a loved one's behavior has us at wit's end, or whether we eat nothing but junk food—the body hangs in there with us, striving for harmony. Many of the adjustments it makes take place while we are asleep, which is why we awaken feeling rejuvenated—and why chronically skimping on sleep is equivalent to dying slowly. The reason we experience the urge to urinate and/or move our bowels immediately upon awakening? Because the body wants to expel all the toxins it mopped up while we slept. Of course, our cells heal themselves better when they have not been damaged by our unproductive lifestyle habits and toxins. The longer we live and eat the standard American diet, the greater a toll it takes on the body. Our cells perform and duplicate themselves less perfectly, leading to aging and disease.

Even for scientists it can be hard to comprehend the countless internal activities our body engages in as it tries to keep us stable. It's easier to imagine ways it does this by looking at activity we can see, so allow me to give you an easy example. Consider what happens if you literally set your body out of balance by leaning too far in one direction. The farther you move away from a vertical and upright position, the more your muscles will clench, your toes grab, and your body adjust to reestablish equilibrium. Lean far enough over and your leg will involuntarily step in the direction you're leaning in an effort to keep you from falling over. It does this without your effort. Of course, you can override that reflexive movement to "catch" yourself, consciously choosing to fall over instead. When we ignore the body's natural instincts, we undermine its effort to keep us in equilibrium. But that's our free will working. The body's natural inclination is to keep us healthy, harmonious, and balanced.

Is Ignorance Bliss?: Ways We Ignore Our Bodies

While it is the body's nature to balance and heal itself, we are able to override many of our natural instincts by exercising our free will. Our society encourages us to mistrust or ignore our bodies, but when we do this, we make ourselves less healthy. Here are some common examples.

Not sleeping when we're tired. Rather than taking an afternoon "siesta" or "power nap" when we're sleepy, many of us reach for stimulants like coffee or caffeinated soda. While most of our ancestors awakened at dawn and went to bed around sundown, we push through our early evening fatigue to stay up to watch the eleven o'clock news. Or we fall asleep, wake ourselves up, then wonder why we're not sleepy when we finally lie down.

Not going to the bathroom. Ignoring the bodily urge to evacuate is a big issue, particularly for women. I cannot tell you how many of my female clients tell me that they go all day without urinating or moving their bowels because they were in a meeting. Not peeing when you need to teaches the bladder muscles to retain more urine than it was designed to. After years of gravity pulling the heavy liquid downward, the bladder muscles become overextended and lose elasticity. No wonder so many mature women develop urinary incontinence. Holding your bowel movements conditions the body not to evacuate the bowels. When this practice is combined with eating denatured foods that the body doesn't know how to digest, you become constipated. Granted, many workplaces don't make it easy to go to the bathroom. It's not unusual for nurses to feel unable to use the bathroom during an entire sixteen-hour double shift, especially in a busy pediatric ward. Many companies give workers only half an hour for lunch and two ten-minute breaks—which not only doesn't leave you much time to take care of your bathroom business, you have to choose between going to the bathroom and calling your kids at home.

Unhealthy practices like these not only train the body to work against its instincts, they cause us to retain toxins in our bodies for longer than nature intended.

Supressing a sneeze. While there's no need to spray your neighbor with germs, it's not a good idea to stop your body from throwing off a toxin the body is violently trying to eject. Sneeze into the crease of your elbow or a tissue instead.

Ignoring a headache. When our temples are throbbing, instead of lying down and figuring out what is making our brain ache, our culture teaches us to take aspirin or Tylenol and keep on stepping. But headaches occur for many reasons, and several of them are severe. Exposure to toxins is one major cause. Many people eat, breathe, or otherwise come into contact with things they are intolerant or allergic to and, consequently, experience headaches. Some people have tension headaches, caused by sluggish blood flow to the brain. These often signal an underlying problem. Some signs can lead to a stroke. Other folks have headaches caused by hormonal imbalances. Still others have brain tumors.

Feeding a fever. Should you starve a cold and feed a fever or feed a cold and starve a fever? Americans are all confused about this time-tested advice. The answer? Listen to your body. A hot fever is created to burn up a virus or bacteria. If you let the fever burn, you'll get rid of the bug by sweating. When you have a fever, you generally do not feel very hungry. When you pop a pill to reduce your temperature, you may feel more like eating, but the "bug" will still be inside you.

Taking an antidiarrheal. When we have the "runs," it's a sign that our body is trying to cleanse a "bug" our out of our bowels. But instead of letting the body purge, many of us take medicines to stop the process. That one leaves me scratching my head. If your body is literally exploding toxins out of you, why in the world would you want to trap the "crap" inside? The answer: Because people don't understand that their body is always working in their best interest.

Overeating. One of the most common ways we override our body's innate intelligence is by misusing food. Clients are constantly telling me that they eat when they're not really hungry. Many of us learn this bad habit during childhood from our well-meaning parents. "But I'm not hungry," you often hear children say—to which your parents often reply, "Eat it anyway!" Other people eat because they're angry, lonely, tired, bored, or sad. Still others tell me, "I just eat when I'm supposed to" or "I just eat everything on my plate." I remind them that even though their parents taught them to eat at 8 A.M., noon, and 6 P.M. or to clear their plate because there are "children starving in Africa," the best thing to do is to eat when you're hungry. For most people, this means consuming a very small meal or snack every two hours or so.

Engaging in recreational eating. There is a difference between productive eating, whose goal is to nourish the body, and recreational eating, which I define as eating solely for taste, because it's dinnertime, for companionship, to celebrate, or because you're stuffing down your emotions. When we eat recreationally, the question we ask ourselves is: "What tastes good?" When we eat productively, we ask ourselves: "What is this going to do for my body?" When we engage in productive eating, we're using our food as our medicine.

The Acid/Fat Connection

You probably didn't realize it at the time, but you learned a lot about body harmony in high school science class. You may remember that you can use a piece of litmus paper to measure an item's *pH* (short for *potential hydrogenation*, a term you rarely see used), an indicator of its acid/alkaline balance. pH is measured on a scale of 1 to 14, with 1 being the most *acidic* reading possible and 14 being the most *alkaline* or *basic*. Stick litmus paper into some soapy water and it will turn blue, reflecting an alkaline pH that falls somewhere between 9 and 10. If you stick litmus paper into vinegar, it will turn golden yellow, indicating its acidity. At 7, pure water is neutral and doesn't change the color of litmus paper at all. However, most Americans live in places where chemicals like fluoride are added to cleanse the water, making our water more acidic than nature intended.

The body's drive to establish equilibrium is reflected in its biochemistry. The pH of the human body should fall anywhere between 6.5 and 7.0. This reading represents the balance between healthy cells, whose pH is more toward the alkaline, and waste products the cells secrete, which are largely acidic. (Your urine should be acidic in the morning because your body has been scrubbing the toxins out overnight.) When we consume a lot of processed foods, take medications, or are under a lot of stress, the body becomes more acidic. For example, the following list shows the approximate pH of some common foods (the values vary depend on the variety of the food, whether it is fresh, canned, or packaged, etc.):

- Apples: 3.5
- Beans: 6.0
- Beef (ground): 5.6
- Beer: 4.4
- Bread: 5.5
- Broccoli: 6.4
- Coffee: 5.0
- Corn: 6.5
- Citrus fruit: 2.3
- Eggs: 7.9
- Fish: 6.7
- Ketchup: 3.9
- Jelly: 3.3
- Mayonnaise: 4.4
- Milk: 6.6
- Oatmeal: 6.4
- Peanut butter: 6.3
- Pork: 6.0
- Salmon: 6.1
- Soda pop: 2.5
- Sugar: 5.5
- Tomatoes: 4.5
- Watermelon: 5.4
- Wine: 3.1

For comparison, consider the pH of some common products:

- Acid rain: 3.5
- Ammonia: 11
- Battery acid: 1
- Bleach: 11
- Blood: 7.4
- Liquid drain cleaner: 14

- Oven cleaner: 12+
- Saliva: 6.7
- Sea water: 7.5 to 8.4
- Stomach acid: 1

- Urine: 4.5 to 8, depending how acidic the person's body is

When we consume a diet containing a variety of vegetables, fruits, nuts and seeds, and lots of vitamins and minerals, the body becomes more alkaline. Because the typical American diet and lifestyle are so out of balance, our pH tends to be very acidic.

While having an overly acidic body doesn't mean you have a disease, it causes you to experience a lower-grade level of living and sets you up to gain weight. When the body is constantly acidic, not enough oxygen is able to flow through our system and our cells get very congested. When our cells can't breathe and are all backed up, we become tired, hyperactive, emotionally unstable, and angrier than we are under more healthy conditions. Some people become very stressed out. When we're stressed, we secrete epinephrine, the hormone that causes the "fight-or-flight" reaction. Epinephrine is very acidic and contributes to the body's being chronically acidic.

When the body's pH is knocked out of equilibrium, we may start craving certain foods, as the body seeks out vitamins and minerals that will help it create homeostasis. Unfortunately, many of us have trained our brain that certain vitamins and minerals it needs are found in processed foods. Most processed foods are also acidic.

If you eat a diet high in refined foods, those are the foods you'll crave: potato chips, ice cream, extra crispy fried chicken, chocolate chip cookies. Unfortunately, some of the foods an acid body craves are also foods that it's allergic to. Again, this is because we've taught it that these foods are where it will find certain nutrients. Since we'll also experience an allergic reaction, eating these foods will actually make us feel worse.

By shifting to a balanced diet containing all the right vitamins, minerals, enzymes, and phytonutrients, an acid body can become more alkaline. As it becomes more alkaline, it immediately begins to produce healthier cells, making us feel better quickly. We can intentionally flush the acid out of the body, helping it achieve equilibrium and making us feel more vibrant, energetic, and peaceful—the body's natural state. As we do this, the body automatically gravitates to a healthy weight—and you don't have to deprive yourself, exercise, or go on a diet.

The Confusion over Calories

The traditional American weight-loss diet encourages people to reduce the number of calories they eat in order to force the body to burn more fat. But there's a fundamental problem with this theory: the body of a *Homo sapiens* (Latin for "wise man" or "knowing man)" absolutely *hates* to burn fat. Why? For over two hundred thousand years, most of our ancestors were hunters and gatherers whose bodies adapted to having abundant amounts of food to eat after an animal was slaughtered or crops were harvested. Their bodies then allowed them to survive scarcity after that food had been consumed. To withstand this environment of literal feast or famine, the human body learned that whenever excess food was available, the body stood a better chance of riding out the inevitable lean months if it learned to convert any extra nutrients into fat. Fat not only kept our forbears warm and cushioned their organs, it stored nutrients the body could call upon to keep them alive during lean times. Given this history, it is literally human nature to store fat for future use. Though food is now plentiful in our society, we need only go back a few generations to see how this instinct to conserve flab helped our ancestors weather crop failures and famines.

With this as the backdrop, let's consider this modern-day activity we call dieting. At its essence, dieting consists of starving our body so it will lose weight. Already, you can see the problem. *Homo sapiens*'s brain is so intelligent, has been fine-tuned for so many millennia, and is so intent on keeping our species alive that it outmaneuvers our dietary strategy of depriving ourselves to shed pounds. We only need to miss a meal or two before a warning alarm is sent out to the cells: "Oh, my goodness! She's starving again. Hang onto every nutrient you can. We have to save her life!" The body then slows down our metabolism, the rate at which we consume nutrients to obtain energy from them, so that it consumes fewer while we're dieting than it does when we're nourishing ourselves properly. Once we end our diet and resume eating normally, our brain outthinks us, telling the body, "I know her by now. It's not going to be long before she starves herself again. Keep metabolizing food slowly and hang on to every nutrient you can. We've got extra room around her middle so stick everything extra onto her belly, thighs, and buttocks so we have a little extra in store for next time."

Women's bodies, in particular, store fat around their middle so food is located close to the fetus should they become pregnant during a famine. After dieting, even if we eat the exact same amount of the exact same foods we ate before we started purging pounds, we're going to put on extra weight. Over time, repeat dieters train their bodies to hold onto more fat every time they try to lighten up. Of course, this is the average person's worst-case scenario. But placed within the context of humankind's struggle to survive scarcity and famine, who can blame our brain for taking our actions so seriously? The human body cannot overcome a quarter of a million years of conditioning in less than seventy-five years!

Adding insult to injury, since the body clings to every bit of food we feed it, it also clings to every toxin that we consume along with it—you know, those artificial flavors and colors, antibiotics, and hormones found in processed foods. The more toxins get stored in the body, the more they congest us, make us feel "off," cause us to lose energy, and, eventually, make us sick. They also contribute to the cellulite that everyone dreads, causing our bottom to jiggle and leading us to start another diet. Now we're caught up in the cycle of rollercoaster weight loss, where we lose pounds only to gain back more weight and toxins.

Notice that as I describe this cycle of yoyoing weight, I am writing about nutrients but not calories. The culture of dieting teaches us that the number of calories we eat determines whether we gain or lose weight. While it is true that you'll gain weight if you eat more calories than you burn off, counting calories is not the answer to everyone's weight-loss dilemma. In fact, it is even possible for the same person to gain more weight by eating fewer calories than they did in the past. How so? One way is to get caught in a cycle of rollercoaster dieting. Another is by eating low-nutrient foods.

While it's rare that we think of calories in terms of anything but weight, they're actually a measure of the amount of potential energy contained within our food. Different types of foods contain different amounts of energy: carbohydrates count four calories per gram; protein offers four calories per gram; and dietary fat weighs in at nine calories per gram. So for all the negative press it gets, dietary fat—that is, the fat you obtain from foods, as opposed to body fat, which you carry on your body—has the potential to give us more energy per gram than any other food. Unfortunately, many people have been misled into believing that because dietary fat contains the most calories, eating it automatically piles on body fat. They also mistakenly believe that reducing dietary fat means you automatically lose weight. In reality, the quality of the food we eat is a major determinant of how much fat the body holds on to and how easily we shed pounds. Food that contains a lot of nutrients gives us more energy than highly processed foods or "junk" foods, so called because they contain little nutrition. Just like your car becomes sluggish and operates inefficiently if you put cheap oil into it, your metabolism becomes lethargic if you eat poor-quality food. Low-quality calories do not burn off at the same rate as high-quality calories. To give you an example: One gram of dietary fat obtained from a low-nutrient, highly processed food like potato chips yields less energy than one gram of dietary fat from a nutrient-dense snack like a rice cake topped with almond butter. The body burns chips less efficiently. As a result, they are more likely to sit on your hips. That's why five hundred calories obtained from a nutrient-dense source can give you more energy and make your metabolism behave more efficiently than a thousand calories from junk food. This is one of the major reasons why big junk-food eaters can often be found sitting on the sofa.

Focusing solely on calories is misguided for other reasons as well. Consider a woman who plays tennis regularly so she has well-toned muscles and a low level of body fat. Because muscles burn more energy than fat, even when she is sitting down, our tennis player will burn more calories than a couch potato or someone ill who doesn't have a lot of muscles and has a higher percentage of body fat. Yet she, too, will react negatively to eating junk food. Feed her a thousand low-nutrient calories and she'll have problems digesting them, feel sluggish, and her energy will drop. But if she eats a thousand nutrient-dense calories, she'll have a lot of energy.

So the number of calories that we eat isn't always as important as either the diet industry or manufacturers of low-calorie foods would like us to think. And the number of nutrients those calories contain is far more important than any manufacturer of processed foods wants you to know. This is just another reason why it is important to eat more whole, nutrient-dense, fresh foods like fruits, vegetables, whole grains, nuts, seeds, fish, poultry, and meats, and to avoid processed and refined foods, which contain the least amount of nutrients and the most toxins. If you do not eat enough food and/or that food does not contain much nutrition in it, not only will you lack stamina, rather than burning the food for energy, your body will slow its metabolism and cling to it for dear life. And where will it get stored? That's right—in your fat cells. If, on the other hand, you feed your body nutrient-dense food, it will shed fat easily and effortlessly and calorie counting will be unnecessary.

Given all of these different factors, it's no wonder that diets don't work! Each and every time we try to lose weight using a strategy that deprives us of nutrients, we swim upstream against the tide of human evolution. Like cutting our hair off, shaving our beard or legs, or trimming our fingernails and hoping they won't grow back, whenever we embark on a diet, we're fighting against human nature!

For a low-calorie approach to weight loss to work, it must feed you high-quality foods that contain a lot of nutrition. Although the concept seems to defy logic, you must eat in order to lose weight!

> **FACTOID**
>
> If you don't provide your body with adequate nutrition, it will hold on to fat for dear life. Give it enough nutrition and it will shed fat and pounds without your even making an effort!

The Pros and Cons of Popular Diets

For many years I counted myself among America's millions of diet kings and queens. As toxic as my body was and as efficiently it held on to weight, I think I went on every diet known to man. I have suffered through the process like everyone else. Following is a summary of what I like and dislike about a number of popular weight-loss approaches, evaluated through the lens of both my personal experience and that of a health care professional.

The Atkins Diet

Pro: Causes people to lose weight quickly.

Con: The brain cannot function normally when fed less than ninety grams of carbohydrates daily, which the Atkins Diet encourages. Because the diet creates high levels of acidity in the body, eating in the manner the Atkins Diet recommends flushes out major minerals, including calcium, magnesium, potassium, and sodium; creates a condition in the body called ketosis, in which fat is being broken down very quickly, which can damage the kidneys; and because you starve yourself of nutrition, Atkins dieters often experience a major weight-gain rebound effect.

Verdict: Don't try it. This diet is very dangerous. It has destroyed many a kidney!

Dr. Bob Arnot's Revolutionary Diet

Pro: This is essentially a therapeutic nutritional plan designed to prevent heart attacks and cancer, especially colon cancer, and appropriately nourish people already diagnosed with chronic diseases, such as diabetes.

Con: The plan is complicated and highly scientific, since the nutritional regime is designed for hospitals to use to treat chronic illnesses such as cancer.

Verdict: This is a good diet for health care professionals to teach their patients suffering from chronic diseases. It's too complicated for the average person to practice every day.

Dr. Shapiro's Picture Perfect Diet

Pros: This very creative book contains photographs of what you should and should not eat, plus over 180 food equations that give readers an abundance of options. Dr. Shapiro dieters can eat in restaurants, as long as they can remember what they should and should not consume.

Cons: This diet offers too much freedom, and dieters have to remember too many plans.

Verdict: When following a diet that allows you the freedom to eat so many foods, you risk unknowingly triggering food allergies that will cause your weight loss to be less successful than it could be.

Eat Right for Your Type

Pros: Eat Right instructs readers to customize their food choices according to their body chemistry, as reflected in their blood type: A, AB, B, or O. Adjusting your diet in the way this book advises makes weight loss easier, eliminates cravings, strengthens your immune system, and combats digestive ailments, fatigue, and allergies.

Con: Restricts you to eating certain foods that are supposedly most compatible with your blood type; however, the four-blood-type nutrition concept is very controversial.

Verdict: There is no genetic or molecular evidence of an association between any specific blood type and a corresponding set of food choices.

Fit for Life Rotation Diet

Pros: This approach involves eating only foods that are in the same food group each day, say, dairy products or meats. For that reason, it's a good diet for people with a weak digestive system and helps to eliminate allergies and food intolerances.

Cons: Has too many constraints. The amount of scientific information it contains is overwhelming.

Verdict: Very limited in its ability to help you keep weight off.

The Glycemic Index

Pros: This book teaches readers to use the glycemic index, a ranking of carbohydrates based on their effect on blood glucose levels, to select the carbs they should eat, thereby helping them to control their weight. Effectively levels blood sugar and causes weight loss.

Cons: Too many numbers, charts, and graphs.

Verdict: Requires too much studying for the average person to succeed with it.

Jenny Craig

Pros: The Jenny Craig diet makes everything practical. Prepacked food eliminates the need to select healthy food at the grocery store, thereby reducing your temptation to purchase unhealthy items. The weekly support that is included with the program provides good motivation.

Cons: The plan is expensive—even discounted meals may cost $21.99 on top of the groceries you have to buy. The fact that the food is prepackaged makes it difficult to share meals with family and friends or to dine out. Some don't like the taste of the food.

Verdict: Too restrictive, so you can't do it for long.

The Perricone Diet

Pro: Dr. Perricone recommends eating foods containing antioxidants, vitamins, and amino acids, and often natural substances rich in antioxidants and foods like brightly colored vegetables, berries, tomatoes, and pineapple, as well as foods rich in essential fatty acids like salmon.

Con: In an ideal world, this diet does work. In reality, only a select few people will have the ability to follow it to the letter. It's strict on calorie intake.

Verdict: It is a great diet for antiaging and resolving appearance- and skin-related issues, but it is not for everyone because of the high carbs and calorie restriction.

The Pritikin Diet

Pro: One of the first books to do a good job of explaining the quality of your food as opposed to quantity. If you like carbs, you'll like Dr. Pritikin's book.

Cons: Requires strict portion control. The diet is high in carbs, which can lead to insulin surges and subsequent cravings. That can lead to rapid weight gain after you complete the diet.

Verdict: It is very restrictive, so you cannot do it for long.

The Raw Foods Diet

Pro: This diet is full of natural enzymes, and you can eat as much as you want and still lose weight. It is very healthy and will prevent disease.

Con: You can eat only raw foods, which is very restricting.

Verdict: Teaching that cooked food is poison is too one-sided—cooking, for instance, kills lethal and harmful bacteria. Too strict for most people to implement.

The South Beach Diet

Pro: Created by a cardiologist, the popular South Beach Diet includes many tasty recipes containing a great balance of the right kinds of fats and carbs.

Cons: Those who are accustomed to carb-rich diets will find it very demanding. It's also low in protein and heavy in fiber.

Verdict: A great way to lose weight initially, but the weight loss slows down after the first phase of diet.

Weight Watchers

Pros: Weight Watchers is a safe diet promoting good eating habits so you can lose weight without starving yourself. Group support helps dieters adhere to the program.

Cons: Because there are so few restrictions and many different food offerings, people have too much freedom to choose, which makes the program difficult to manage. Many people end up eating everything because it becomes way too complicated. Many people say weight loss is too slow; others hate going to weekly meetings, especially during those times when they're not losing weight.

Verdict: Dieters lose weight too slowly and eventually lose interest.

The Zone

Pros: This diet promotes mindful eating and portion control and regulates sugar intake, normalizing insulin levels. Zone dieters are encouraged to use omega-3 and omega-6 monosaturated fats, obtained from fish, cereals, whole grains, poultry, and eggs, and to avoid trans fats, commonly found in fast and processed foods. Dieters who stick to these guidelines will experience more energy and greater mental clarity.

Cons: The Zone is a calorie-restricted diet that starves the body, setting it up to gain weight later. Its dietary rules are very complicated to follow and almost impossible to maintain. Plus, the diet promotes eating too much protein, causing the body to become overly acidic.

Verdict: Very low in carbohydrates and is too restrictive.

Detoxing Differs from Dieting

When we consistently provide the body with good nutrition, the brain no longer believes the body is dieting, so it chills out and stops telling the body to hold on to fat. This is the difference between diets of good nutrition like South Beach and Perricone, which work, and starvation diets like Atkins and Pritikin, where you're destined to gain weight back. When we nourish our bodies well, the excess fat the body has stored is released and a boatload of toxins along with it, helping you to feel better and actually become healthier. Provided with enough nutrition, it even uses the nutrients to repair damaged cells. All of this happens very quickly, effortlessly, and naturally. You don't have to eat a lot of grapefruit, drink yet another weight-loss shake, or even join a gym.

Detoxing differs from dieting in that its goal is to cleanse and rest the body. However, one of the natural consequences of detoxing is that excess weight falls off. Yet, the approaches to the two processes are different. My grandmother knew that flushing harmful substances out of the body keeps it from getting sick. This type of indigenous knowledge has been practiced in every culture, as humans naturally understood the importance of cleansing from the inside out. If you go back just a couple of generations, you'll find that many of our forbears employed some method of cleansing their vital organs. These practices are still common in less industrialized countries, where you'll find people using herbs like *aloe vera* or *cascara sagrada* or bush (also called Zulu) or senna tea to regularly cleanse their bodies. Today, many kinds of detoxification programs are used in the industrialized world. Of course, we're all familiar with detoxes that cleanse people of the negative effects of drugs and alcohol. Yet you can also help your body expel toxins that have gotten trapped in the cells and organs from being exposed to noxious elements in our environment and food. There are many types of nutritional detoxification programs. While their goals vary, they generally aim to stop the digestive process to allow the body to purge poisons and revitalize itself.

Fasting

Popular during the 1960s and 1970s, the practice is now outdated and the term often used very loosely—some people say they're "fasting" from shopping or lifestyle excesses. The goals of fasting vary from depriving yourself for spiritual reasons to resting the digestive tract and cleansing the body. People may fast by consuming only water, or water with lemon juice or apple cider vinegar. The "Master Cleanse" fast, consisting of water, lemon juice, maple syrup, and cayenne pepper, goes in and out of vogue.

But while fasting may have been healthy during a simpler time, fasting today can make us very sick. For example, we all have DDT—a very virulent pesticide that is now illegal in the United States, although it is used many places overseas—stored in our fat. Fasts—and particularly water fasts—dump deadly chemicals like DDT out of our fat and into our bloodstream more quickly than our liver may be able to endure. Fasting also provides little to no nutrition, putting most Americans at risk of serious illness, since so many of us are either already or borderline malnourished.

Detoxification or Cleansing Detox

Detoxes help the body move closer to equilibrium by helping it purge mental, emotional, environmental, water, and food toxins while simultaneously resting the digestive system. I believe that, unfortunately, every American needs to detox—that's what terrible shape we're all in these days. People detox themselves in many ways, including by reducing or eliminating red meat or fast or junk foods from their diet, eating as a vegetarian, consuming only fresh fruit or vegetable juices. Many people detox for as little as one day. The most effective detox programs include nutritional supplements that nourish the cells as they release excess waste. Fresh juice detoxes are an example of this. When we detox, we release pent-up emotions as well; for as the body releases waste, it also releases emotions whose biochemistry was stored alongside the toxins because, say, we ate a box of donuts because we're sad rather than just crying, journaling, or making a structural change that would relieve our sadness.

Cleansing Diet Detox

A cleansing diet detox cleans out the body by providing it with maximum nutrition in small doses. This approach allows the body to release toxins and, along with it, excess weight. Because the

---

FAQ: Is Detoxing Dangerous?

Q: My doctor claims that we don't need to detox because the body is equipped to detoxify itself. He says it isn't safe. Is he right?

A: Actually, your doctor is partially right—but he's lacking some vital information. It is true that detoxing can be dangerous. As I noted above, fasting—especially water fasts—can be very harmful, because they cause massive amounts of dangerous toxins to be dumped into the bloodstream very, very quickly. Depending on a host of factors ranging from how healthy you are to how nutritionally you eat to what kinds of toxins your body contains, someone who participates in a fast could become very, very sick.

It's important to detoxify at a rate your body can healthily withstand, and to nourish the body to help it repair the parts of it that the toxins have injured. Detox programs that include a rebuilding component such as fresh vegetable juices are much healthier than those involving water or some variation of water and lemon juice. Every detox program and person is different, so I agree with your doctor in that I cannot vouch that these kinds of programs will be absolutely safe given your specific health conditions.

But here's where your doctor's explanation comes up short: the body is equipped with eliminatory organs that work perfectly in an unpolluted environment where people eat nutrient-dense whole (unprocessed) foods. Americans don't do that. To stay healthy or even to manage or heal from our illnesses, we have to cleanse our systems. We can do this in a variety of ways, ranging from nutritional detoxes to colon hydrotherapy (colonics) to coffee enemas to lymph drainage massages. These types of interventions are necessary if we are to experience optimal health. When we detoxify in a way that not only cleanses but also rebuilds damaged tissues and cells, detoxifying is not only very safe, but it's also a quick-healing strategy that can be used by even the sickest human being.

---

body receives sufficient nutrition, it does not experience a "yo-yo" back up to its previous weight once the detox has been completed. The Martha's Vineyard Detox is a cleansing detox. It provides maximum nutrition in forms that help it rapidly heal visible and invisible damage to body organs and tissues.

Testimonial

MARCIA BUCKLEY

Age: 61
Occupation: pastor
Location: Martha's Vineyard, Massachusetts

I have known Dr. Roni for a number of years; I pastor her church, Martha's Vineyard Apostolic House of Prayer. During the time we've been acquainted, I have gained a lot of weight. At my heaviest I was at least 100 pounds overweight. I tried to get my weight down for a long, long time. At one point I lost as much as 65 or 70 pounds. But each time I lost weight, I would put more back on. The more diets I tried, the bigger I got. Dr. Roni witnessed some of my struggles. At one point she invited me to the Inn to try her program. To tell you the truth, I wasn't keen on detoxing or those kinds of things—in fact, I wasn't really aware of what it meant—so I brushed her off.

In the meantime I started having health problems. I kept experiencing different aches and pains. I started getting sick a lot. I couldn't go up the stairs or even work without becoming winded. A couple of years earlier, I had become a grandmother and was so weighed down by all this weight I was dragging around that I had begun wondering, "How am I going to keep up with this little girl?" My daughter was really worried about me. My blood pressure was high, so I had to go on medication. At one point I felt like I was having heart problems. Fortunately, they couldn't find anything wrong with it, but every time I went to the hospital for a checkup, they told me I needed to lose weight. Needless to say, all these changes were very frightening to me. But I also started asking myself, "What kind of example am I as a pastor?" I knew I wasn't a very good witness to those I was speaking to about taking care of their bodies and health.

At some point during my struggles, James Hester had started coming to the church. I knew that he had completed the detox and had done really well, as had several of the friends he had brought to the island. One day James told me, "Next week, I'm going to do the detox again. Why don't you do it with me?" I thought, "Well, that gives me a week to prepare myself." So I just made up my mind, "That's it; I'm going to do it." Even though I had avoided the program for years, when I went into it I was very positive. I don't like to do anything that I don't believe in wholeheartedly. My goals were to lose weight and improve my health. I expected everything to happen just like James said—that I'd lose 21 pounds in 21 days.

I had a good time doing the detox. I really enjoyed it, to be honest. Knowing that I was accomplishing something that I should have been doing for myself all along felt really good. Dr. Roni had warned me that I was going to get tired and would have to rest, but that never really happened. Between eating all those vegetables and taking the supplements, I might have gotten a little tired one day, but I mainly became a lot more energetic. One thing that I noticed right away was that my face turned several shades lighter. It was like all the toxins and things that weren't supposed to be in my body were causing all this darkness in my skin. I have "before" and "after" pictures of myself, and while the fact that I lost weight is really obvious, the other thing you notice is the brightness in my skin. And I was getting so many compliments from everybody, I knew I had to stick with it.

Several weeks into the detox, I noticed that my blood pressure had gone way down and the medication I had been taking was starting to make me feel strange. I talked to my sister, who's a nurse, and she suggested that I cut my dose a little bit every other day. I did that, but the medication still made me feel lightheaded. So I thought, "Let me see how I do without taking it at all." I didn't take my medication for a couple of days; yet, I felt better and my pressure stayed down. Dr. Roni warned me to be very careful, but I decided to step out on faith and stop taking my medicine. To this day, my blood pressure is normal. Also while I was detoxing my thinking became clearer and I drew closer to the Lord. More parishioners suddenly started complimenting my sermons. I'm still not certain what happened, but you know the saying "healthy, wealthy and wise"? Well, I think that as I became healthier I also gained more wisdom.

The only difficult thing that happened was that I began to experience pain in my knee. I broke my ankle a few years ago, and the knee on that leg has stayed weak. When I was going through the process and the toxins started coming out, my knee became very painful and

I had to go back on crutches for about a week. I was very upset until Dr. Roni explained that I was experiencing a healing crisis and that the toxins were coming out through the weak point in my body.

"If you can stand the pain, just go through it," she said. "It's going to be all right."

And she was right. After about a week the pain subsided. But that was the worst part because it felt like I was going backwards, though I learned that I really wasn't. I also felt chilled a couple of times, which, I guess, is part of the process. But those were things I'd expected. That was the extent of my healing crisis.

Things went so well that I ended up detoxing twice. The first time, I lost about 22 to 23 pounds. I was so excited! Because it was healthy, this approach seemed to answer to a lot of the problems I'd had in the past with other diets! It wasn't just going on a diet and stopping this and stopping that, then eating again and putting it back on. This program offered a way that I could eat healthily for the rest of my life. I wanted to keep going past the 21 days, but Dr. Roni told me I needed protein. So I stopped and ate some protein and healthy foods for a few weeks. When it was safe, I went right back on the program again. Between the two detoxes, I lost almost 50 pounds!

When my daughter saw how good I looked, she tried the program herself. So did my sister and son-in-law. It was like a chain reaction happened—it was kind of contagious! Everyone saw me and thought, "Wow! You look good. I've got to do this." Several of my church members went on the program, and a few more just got colonics. I loved it! My success was affecting everybody. I even put the church on a 21-day Daniel fast, where they would eat fruits and vegetables, brown rice, nuts, and beans. No preservatives, no sugar, no sweetened juices. Everyone was reading labels. They were very good about it. We all looked and felt better and had a great time.

Even though I gained back some of the weight, I still felt younger—I feel thirty-five years old. I'm able to be more active and keep up with my granddaughter. I joined a gym, so I actually work out now. I also ride my stationary bike at home. And even though my weight is slightly up from where it was, I'm still off the blood pressure medication.

3

THE MARTHA'S VINEYARD DIET DETOX

Reduce, Rejuvenate, and Rebuild

In August 2003, I went on a vacation in Mexico to give myself a summer break, something I rarely do because it's peak season on the Vineyard. I had been burning the candles at both ends helping other people to heal and needed to take some time to take care of myself. I booked myself into a private home where I planned to do a detox. I also intended to travel around the country to obtain a number of cleansing and healing treatments under Dr. Martinez's care. One day while he was treating me, Dr. Martinez told me he wanted to examine my stool to determine if I had parasites. Parasites?! I knew the statistics—one in three Americans' bodies harbors them. But being a healer, I didn't want it to be me.

"But I've been eating healthy," I protested when the test came back positive. "I've only been eating vegetables."

"Those must have been some very good vegetables," he answered.

I have to tell the truth: I was upset. No one likes to consider the thought that their body might be a home to parasites—especially not a healer. And who wants to think too much about their colon, never mind what's in it?

"Fortunately, you have a parasite that's easy to get rid of," Dr.

Martinez told me. He gave me a very common allopathic medication called Iodiquinol. Unbeknownst to him, I did not take it. I waited until I returned to Martha's Vineyard and ordered a parasite cleanse, containing herbal-based products such as black walnut, wormwood, mugwort, and cloves, that I use at my retreat. I also took an herbal tea whose ingredients clean and repair the lining of the digestive tract and remove parasites and debris from the body. I took the parasite cleanse for 45 days; some protocols are longer, others are shorter. Either way, parasites are difficult to get rid of. I still drink a special Indian tea that tastes really good and keeps me from getting parasites again (see recipe on page 183).

Although we often associate parasites with unsanitary conditions, dirty drinking water, and undeveloped nations, they're alive and well all over the world. We get them when we globetrot; they can jet over to our supermarket atop imported food and float in by way of our drinking water. When I have a client who constantly feels bloated; is always hungry; experiences chronic nausea, forgetfulness, fatigue, slow reflexes, or sexual dysfunction; or can't lose weight, I test them for parasites right away. Sadly, most American doctors are not knowledgeable about parasites. If you have any of the above symptoms, tell your doctor you are concerned that you have them or order a parasite test kit to be delivered to your home (www.mvdietdetox.com).

What Is the Martha's Vineyard Diet Detox?

Parasites are one of many toxins and foreign substances that can interfere with our metabolism and cause us to gain weight and have a hard time taking it off. I have scientifically formulated the Martha's Vineyard Diet Detox to cleanse the body of many of the poisons posing the greatest risk to our health, including toxins in these six categories:

1. Food toxins, including artificial flavors, colors, preservatives, excess sodium, antibiotics, hormones, and pesticides
2. Toxins already in our body, including those from mercury dental fillings as well as the mercury found in some childhood

vaccines, and residue that remains in our cells after taking over-the-counter and prescription drugs

3. Household toxins, such as chemicals found in cleaning products

4. Water toxins: the chlorine and fluoride in our drinking water, as well as the residue from other people's prescription drugs

5. Environmental toxins, such as air pollution and lawn pesticides

6. Toxins in personal-care products like makeup, cosmetics, shampoos, and deodorants

As your body conducts this housekeeping, you will naturally lose weight. There are also ways to tweak the Diet Detox to help you kill parasites and help improve, perhaps even heal, some chronic health conditions, such as diabetes and hypertension.

The Martha's Vineyard Diet Detox causes the body to conduct two activities. First, it stimulates the cells to cleanse themselves and flush toxins out of the body. It also creates conditions in the body that cause it to repair damaged cells quickly. We spur the body to engage in these activities by doing three things:

1. **Eating maximum nutrition in small doses.** By maximum nutrition, I mean that you will receive a minimum of twenty-two servings of fruits and vegetables daily in modest servings of soups, fresh live juices, and supplements. Compare this to the five to nine servings per day the U.S. Department of Agriculture (USDA) recommends. According to the USDA, the average American gets 1.4 servings of fruit and 3.7 servings of veggies, for a total of 5.1 servings daily (www.mvdietdetox .com).

2. **Nourishing yourself about every two hours—sooner if you get hungry.** Rather than starving your body, being hungry, and later experiencing the yo-yo effect—or, conversely, eating large meals containing excess calories that the body converts to fat—you'll eat only what your body can burn off in a two-hour period of time. Then you'll eat again.

3. **Consuming your nutrients in liquid form.** When we don't chew, our digestive system can rest. When the digestive system is asleep, the energy that the body would normally spend metabolizing food is freed up and available to engage in some R&R: repair and rebuilding! (www.mvdietdetox.com)

Because your body will download toxins into your organs very quickly, you will need to act aggressively to get them out of your body. This means you'll need to drink plenty of water to rinse out the cells, go walking, and engage in specific activities to get the poisons out of your colon, liver, kidneys, lymph system, gallbladder, and skin. I'll explain these processes in greater detail in

---

Water, Water Everywhere—But Which One Should I Drink?

Similar to our planet Earth, over two-thirds of the human body is composed of water. The role of water is to clean and flush the body. Sadly, most of the water we drink is no longer very pure. If it hasn't been treated with fluoride or other toxins at the local water treatment plant, it often contains hard minerals—mainly calcium and magnesium—that have seeped into the water while it was still underground. This is particularly true of tap water, which is one reason why so many people buy bottled. Hard minerals deposit harmful residue in the body that corrodes our smooth tissues, a type of cells found in walls of organs, arteries, and veins. No wonder bottled water sales are booming! But bottled water is usually packaged in plastic, and we now know that chemicals from plastic bottles "out-gas"—disperse in gaseous form—into the environment, which is one reason we shouldn't microwave Styrofoam or plastic wrap.

For detoxing, I prefer distilled water. Distilled water has been boiled and its steam recondensed back into water in a clean container, leaving contaminants and impurities like hard minerals behind. Of course, distilled water isn't really that pure if it's been bottled in plastic, which is why for detoxing I suggest you distill your water at home. In reality, I know most people aren't going to do that. A distilling machine costs between $99 and $299 or more but only cleans the water one drop at a time, yielding about one gallon of water overnight. Many people drink a lot more water than that, especially if they have a family. So there are really no great options. Still, during the detox I'd like you to drink distilled water of one type or another—ideally that you treat yourself, but not in plastic jugs. After your detox is over, unless you continue taking supplements and juicing, return to spring water in jugs to make sure you get your minerals.

Chapter 6. Cleansing these organs also helps protect us against our genetic weak links that get triggered when toxins injure us, causing us to suffer from diseases like breast cancer, colon cancer, liver cancer, diabetes, and heart disease.

Stage One: The Cleanup

The cleansing phase of the Detox stimulates the body to download toxins that have been stored in its fat cells and organs into your bloodstream. The blood then carries these toxins to the eliminatory organs—the colon, liver, and kidneys—so that those organs can expel them. We stimulate the body to engage in this type of spring cleaning by consuming large amounts of fresh vegetables, particularly green ones. Most of the food groups—fruits, starches, grains, beans, nuts, seeds, and fats—build our cells. Vegetables contain nutrients that cleanse them. Green vegetables are particularly purifying. Nature provides us with countless examples of this green-cleaning phenomenon. Trees help cleanse the air, which is why scientists around the world are worried about deforestation. Our pets vomit after eating grass. While we often look at vomiting as a bad thing and believe our pet ate the grass because he doesn't know better, we couldn't be more mistaken. Our pet knew that he needed to expel a "bug" or other toxin from his body and that eating grass would help him throw up. Before companies started marketing aromatherapy household cleansers, many cleaners were pine scented. Tea-tree oil is another popular cleaning product, particularly if you shop in health-food stores. Green things are the equivalent of nature's mop. That's why they're vital to the Martha's Vineyard Diet Detox.

We'll supplement our fresh vegetables by taking nutrient-dense, food-based nutritional supplements. I'm not talking about the vitamins comprised of synthetic chemicals that are sold in most supermarkets and drug and health-food stores. When you take vitamins comprised of man-made substances, you need only look at your fluorescent urine to see the evidence that your body cannot process some of the chemicals. Instead, you'll consume nutritional supplements derived from food sources since the body can more effectively metabolize their nutrients. We will use supplements whose nutrient load is especially dense (www.mvdiet detox.com).

Because the Martha's Vineyard Diet Detox exceeds your daily nutritional needs, the brain stops obsessing about whether your body has adequate nutrients and not only sheds harmful toxins but also the fat that houses them. And since the body isn't being starved, there's no rebound effect!

Stage Two: Repair and Rebuild

The second objective of the Martha's Vineyard Diet Detox is healing whatever's wrong with your body. There are two aspects of the Detox that support this physical "makeover." First, everything you ingest will be in liquid form—nutritional drinks, liquid supplements, vegetable soups, broths, and fresh juices. During the Diet Detox you will avoid food that you chew. While not chewing may seem counterintuitive—even unnatural—it is a particularly important part of the process. Digesting food requires more energy than any other bodily function. You already know this intuitively. Who doesn't get drowsy after gorging themselves on a big Thanksgiving dinner? When we eat too much, we go to sleep. This is one reason why people who overeat almost always have low energy. When we consume food in liquid form, the body doesn't have to work as hard to break it down, so feeding the cells becomes much more efficient.

Because the body doesn't have to work as hard, when you don't chew, your energy shoots through the roof! Many of my clients tell me they've gained so much energy it feels like they've turned back the clock. Folks who normally lean on the snooze button start popping out of bed or begin facing their day without their usual morning latte. Others no longer feel like they need an afternoon nap or want to fall out when they get home. Even if you are very sedentary or heavy, you may suddenly feel up to working out. Rather than winding down in the evening, you may well feel wide awake until your head hits the pillow, at which point you'll probably rest well.

Not chewing also speeds up healing. The body's innate intelligence directs all the extra nutrients you're consuming all around your body and uses some of that extra energy to help heal your organs and tissues. And here's a really amazing fact: it heals damaged areas in priority order. Some changes—like your skin—will be visible to the naked eye; others will take place in parts of your body you don't even know exist. No wonder sick people that are fed a diet of fresh, raw juices often heal very quickly.

The second way you'll help your body repair itself is by drinking a nutritional supplement that's high in antioxidants. From beta-carotene to lycopene to vitamin E, antioxidants repair cellular damage, make us look younger, and help prevent chronic illnesses like heart disease and cancer. Antioxidants act as the body's housekeepers, sweeping up dangerous free radicals, very unstable molecules that can interfere with cellular function. The body creates some antioxidants naturally; others it gets from food.

Though we usually hear about free radicals being dangerous, the body benefits by having some. For instance, the immune system sometimes creates them to help "mop up" viruses and bacteria. And our body is always sloughing off old cells and replacing them with new ones. Free radicals are created during that process. But stress, pollution, cigarette smoke, herbicides, pesticides, and other toxins create more free radicals than our body is supposed to carry. Once altered by free radicals, good cells mutate and interfere with the function of others, setting off a chain reaction of cells running amok. Instead of carrying out their normal function, these cells corrode the body and cause it to "rust." Unchecked, they attack and damage our delicate membranes. The damage free radicals cause is visible in the form of wrinkles, age spots, dry skin, and tired-looking eyes, for example. Inside the body, the injuries range from the body simply breaking down to experiencing a heart attack or stroke. Free radicals can also assault our DNA, causing it to create cancer cells.

Antioxidants help put free radicals in check and keep them from damaging other cells. When we see someone aging "gracefully," it is generally because they have higher levels of antioxidants than other people in their age group—not that you're supposed to

Why Detoxing Is Antiaging

Throw out the conventional wisdom that wrinkles, Alzheimer's, and aches and pains are an inevitable consequence of growing older! What our society has labeled as aging is actually a body overtaxed with toxins. You show me a tired, achy, and overweight body, and I'll show you someone laboring under the weight of high levels of harmful substances. Flush out the unhealthy chemicals and put good nutrition into the body and it will create millions and millions of revitalized cells. Within days of starting the Martha's Vineyard Diet Detox, you will look and feel like a new person.

One of the first places you'll see these changes is in the quality of your skin. As our protective coating and the body's largest organ, our skin is constantly being assaulted by exhaust fumes, dust created by man-made materials, and toxic chemicals. Too much sun and extreme temperatures create additional stress. Plus, the beauty industry has conditioned us to believe we need "revitalizing" serums and "antiaging" creams. Unfortunately, some of those products actually make the skin less healthy by placing a load of synthetic chemicals into the pores that make the skin breathe in and excrete harmful substances. The polluted water and synthetic soap we wash with only make matters worse.

While you're detoxing, your skin will become very vibrant within just a few days. Detoxifying unclogs those pores, helping the body to secrete poisons, air itself out, and create fresh skin. Many clients discover that the Martha's Vinyard Diet Detox removes years from their face, fading age spots, eliminating wrinkles, and restoring the dewiness of their youth! On the inside of your body, your cells are being rejuvenated as well, causing your cells and organs to function better and areas that have been damaged or injured to be repaired.

look bad as you age, as we've been led to believe. If you take good care of yourself and detoxify regularly, your age will not correlate to the state of physical, mental, and emotional decline common among your same-aged peers.

While vegetables are the food group that cleans up toxins, fruit, especially berries, scoop up free radicals and repair "rust" the best. We will take a high-density antioxidant drink made primarily from berries to spur the body to repair itself very quickly. Depending on the brand you choose, one serving of an antioxidant berry drink may provide the equivalent nutrition of six to ten one-cup servings of berries—which is more than you could eat if you gorged yourself, minus the downside of the excess sugar, which would turn into fat because the body could not digest it fast enough. Berries are also fabulous sources of phytonutrients, which research suggests help stop cancer from developing (www. mvdietdetox.com).

Riding Out the Healing Crisis

As the body cleans house, it dumps toxic residues that have built up in its cells—free radicals, hard minerals, oxidized pollutants from smoke and fumes, herbicides, insecticides, food additives, and even cholesterol, for example—into the bloodstream and organs. This may cause you to feel temporarily under the weather, even sick, and is referred to as a *healing crisis*. Depending on which and how many toxins your body secretes and how quickly it unloads them, your first healing crisis will probably happen between the fourth and sixth day and last from one to three days. During this time you may experience such reactions as acne, rashes, nausea, headaches, sleepiness, fatigue, constipation, diarrhea, runny nose, ear problems, and body aches. If you were chronically ill when you began your detox, your healing crisis may even last for a week or so. For a few days you may actually feel more uncomfortable than you did before you began your cleanse. In fact, it's not unusual for the symptoms of a healing crisis to mimic your chronic illness, since your cells are kicking out the toxins that helped make you sick in the first place.

Another cause of the healing crisis is our cells' resistance to change. Over time, through our lifestyle choices we train our cells to behave in ways that may range from being healthy and clean to toxic and sick. Just like we sometimes have a hard time adapting to our doctor's recommendation that we improve our eating habits, our cells may momentarily dig in their heels when challenged to become more healthful. Don't worry. Before long they will be unable to resist the high-quality nutrition you're feeding them, and will eventually relax and give in. So even though during a healing crisis you may temporarily feel worse, feeling bad is actually a pit stop along the journey toward feeling much, much better.

To minimize the effect that these downloading toxins have on your mind, body, and spirit, in Chapter 6 I recommend a very specific program to help you move those toxins out of your body quickly. Drinking more water will be vitally important. I'll also suggest other cleansing techniques, from colonics to exercising to bathing.

Flushing Out Emotions

I once detoxed a man I'll call Robert, whose wife had divorced him and taken his children to another state. Not surprisingly, Robert was very depressed. Food became his only pleasure, so he overindulged and packed on pounds—200 in about two years. Robert weighed almost 400 pounds when we started working together. The highly concentrated nutrients he took helped his nervous system decrease his depression without pharmaceutical drugs. As his thinking became clearer and he learned about healthy eating, he realized that instead of eating for nourishment, he had been using food to medicate himself and "take the edge off" his deep grief. It dawned on him that by overeating at such a rapid rate he was basically committing suicide. Once Robert understood what was happening, he sought counseling to help him express his sadness more healthily. Today, 150 pounds lighter, Robert feels much better. He understands the power of nutrients, so he no longer feeds his body plastic food. All the changes in his body helped him not just to lose weight but to alter the way he was thinking.

In addition to creating a more pristine body, detoxing purifies your mind, emotions, and spirit. Through the mind/body/spirit connection, as you flush out physical poisons, you'll "hose down" these areas, too. During the first few days of your detox, you may find yourself feeling cheerful and in a great mood. Early-stage detoxers often tell me that they love me. "You just *think* you love me," I laugh. I know that in a few days they may find themselves feeling angry, grumpy, guilty, or sad. Many detoxers experience a phase when they can't stop thinking mean and funky thoughts or want to bite someone's head off. This is normal. It's impossible to engage in physical housecleaning and not do an emotional mop-up.

Although most of us are not aware of it, our cells hold memories, including the biochemistry of our unexpressed thoughts and feelings. While our emotional baggage is locked up in our cells, we feel angry, anxious, hyper, and panicked all the time. When we detox, our cells release these chemicals and your feelings will surface. It's important to allow yourself to experience and express them. Laugh, cry, scream, get angry, become grateful. Journal or draw or sing or pray or write poetry to help whisk them out. Your emotions will subside if you engage them. As they do, you'll feel less of an urge to eat. If you don't express these feelings as they bubble up, you will have cleansed your body but not your thoughts, emotions, or spirit. They will be out of "sync" with the "new you" you've created and unable to sustain the changes you've made. And what's the point in losing weight if you're only going to stuff down the emotions that caused you to overeat in the first place? There's nothing more disheartening than to gain back the weight you just lost.

By Day 21 you'll find yourself feeling calmer, happier, more optimistic and energetic. Because your body has released toxins and millions of fresh new cells have replaced the old unhealthy ones, your body, mind, and spirit will be biologically and biochemically different. You will have set down a lot of the baggage you've been carrying around. You will literally be a different person, right down to your cells.

There is one quick caution I must offer: if you've experienced life traumas such as being raped, molested, or physically abused that you haven't addressed by getting counseling or doing other types of emotional healing, any suppressed emotions will come flooding up. If you are aware that you've experienced these kinds of traumatic life challenges, I suggest that you plan to see a therapist while you detox. That way you'll have support in place when any thoughts and feelings you've stuffed down come bubbling up.

Day by Day: What to Expect

As you begin the Martha's Vineyard Diet Detox, you may be wondering how quickly you will lose weight and experience some of the physical, mental, and spiritual results I've described. Everyone is unique, so your experience will vary. But here's what many MV detoxers tell me they experience.

Days 1–3

Physically: Detoxers lose a few pounds, feel lighter and less exhausted. Most people no longer feel gassy and bloated. Their stomach problems are resolving, and they are going to the bathroom more easily and often.

Mentally: People start thinking more clearly and concentrating better. Their anxiety begins to wane and they get excited about improving their health and losing weight.

Spiritually: The stress of starting the program is over. People feel more relaxed and optimistic.

Days 3–7

Physically: By the end of the first week, detoxers have lost at least 5 pounds. They may feel tired, achy, and fluish; get a headache; and develop a rash or pimples. All of these are signs of a healing crisis—that the body is discharging toxins and fat—and should be welcomed, not feared. During this time the detoxer may need to rest more. It is important to stay true to yourself at this time and not try to please others.

Mentally: As the body releases toxins into the bloodstream, detoxers start to feel the effects. Their minds will probably feel foggy and may struggle to make decisions. This foggy effect is temporary. We call this a healing crisis: feeling worse before you get better.

Spiritually: Most Martha's Vineyard Diet detoxers feel happier, more relaxed, and confident of the plan's effectiveness. Other detoxers will become tearful or sad. They are experiencing an emotional release, which will pass quickly as they move into the second week.

Days 7–10

Physically: The average detoxer has lost roughly 7 to 10 pounds, although some have lost more inches than weight, particularly if they are middle-aged. Still, the weight loss is visible to their friends and family. They are starting to look younger.

Mentally: By now you have begun to master the concepts behind the detox and have started believing you can complete it. At this point many detoxers start striving to live healthier and research more information on the subject.

Spiritually: You feel relieved and want to feel even healthier and happier. After the first week, detoxers pay more attention to themselves, changing things like hairstyles, their way of dress, and how they decorate their surroundings.

Days 11–14

Physically: By Day 14, detoxers see a big difference in the mirror and they like what they see. The waistline, belly, and thighs are shrinking and look thinner. The face looks different because there is a loss of inches in the face and neck. The body feels freer, with better range of motion. Many detoxers say they can breathe better. You stop weighing yourself and are no longer preoccupied with the scale because you know you are losing weight. You have a tremendous amount of energy. You enjoy exercise now.

Mentally: During the middle stage of the MV Detox, people are becoming acquainted with new health knowledge as it applies to their body. Their memory improves, as do their senses of smell and hearing. Decision making is easier, and they want to make changes in their life. During these days many of my detoxers talk about wanting to move to Martha's Vineyard.

Spiritually: People feel calmer, more energetic, and more optimistic and self-confident in their daily life and work. Detoxers also start feeling more spiritual. Many begin a period of deep reflection, during which they become comfortable with silence.

Day 15–17

Physically: By this point the detoxer has lost 15 to 17 pounds or more, and it is obvious to the people around them. They are lighter, their body posture has improved, their skin is smoother and healthier, and their eyes are much brighter. Not surprisingly, they feel much more energetic and can move their bodies faster. Around this time, many detoxers feel more athletic and sports oriented and have a desire to exercise. They can now see dramatic changes compared to their pre-detox habits.

Mentally: People are definitely much clearer thinking and are able to solve problems more quickly and multitask. They are also much more creative and optimistic about future goals.

Spiritually: Detoxers literally see the world through new eyes and have a new approach to life. They are more eager to read books, especially about the body. The spirit is calmer and slower to anger. They start taking delight in their observations, which are sharper.

Days 18–21

Physically: The person has lost roughly 21 pounds and their appearance is leaner and more youthful. The face definitely shows signs of vibrancy, and the posture appears to be erect and poised. Their aches and pains are gone.

Mentally: This person is now at a higher level of thinking, is able to read books more quickly, and tends to be interested and intensely involved in their overall health. They have a keen interest in developing new skills.

Spiritually: As the detox winds down, people feel much happier, very creative, and optimistic about the future. They are making spiritual as well as physical changes in their lives. They are now making better life decisions. Their personality is visibly more peaceful and tranquil.

Connecting with Your Higher Self

"I've had heart palpitations for a year now but didn't know what they were," one of my patients confessed to me. I suggested that she see the doctor right away. Too distracted to make the appointment, she experienced "the Big One"—a heart attack—and was forced to implement lifestyle changes she could have made voluntarily. Another client once told me, "I know that when I get angry my body gets hot," not realizing he was experiencing a classic signal that his blood pressure had gone sky high (*note*: not everyone experiences this symptom of hypertension). Another client walked around with a noticeable tumor in her breast for five years without seeking medical help.

Many Americans are so stressed out, distracted, scared, and preoccupied that they ignore symptoms that should send them running to the emergency room. While our society keeps us out of touch with our body, emotion, and spirit, detoxing helps us reconnect with ourselves. As detoxers flush out the chemistry associated with angry, sad, and anxious thoughts, they often find themselves appreciating people more, noticing the beauty of nature, or even perceiving things that they normally don't notice. Often, on about Day 10 or 11 people tell me, "Wow! I went on this walk and I saw a beautiful butterfly!" I take that as a sign that their cleansing is proceeding perfectly and they are reconnecting with their spirit.

While on the Diet Detox, many people learn for the first time what it is really like to take care of themselves. They realize how badly they need to disengage from some of their normal activities. Once they get used to slowing down and focusing on themselves, many people get a peek into the peaceful lifestyle they can have and the person they can become—and like it! I have had clients radically revamp their lives, start a business they've always

---

The Problem with Salt

I had never seen so much salt in one person's house in my life until I opened my client Jocelyn's spice cupboard. She had table salt, seasoning salt, garlic salt, onion salt, celery salt—you name a kind of salt and she had it! During the 21 days I lived in her home, I called her the Queen of Salt. So it was no surprise to me that Jocelyn also had high blood pressure, her ankles were always swollen, and she was taking medicine for edema—fluid retention.

When we started on the detox, I told her I would be taking her off salt. "How am I going to season my food without it?" she worried. Well, I'll be the first person to 'fess up that when you've been OD'ing on salt, going without it takes some getting used to. But by Day 3 Jocelyn noticed something that amazed her. "Never in my whole life have I seen my ankles when they weren't swollen."

Americans are in a lot of trouble because we've been conditioned to season our food with so much salt. In addition to what we sprinkle atop our plate, sodium is used with other chemicals as a type of preservative in many processed foods. It's also added to mask the lack of flavor remaining after refining strips out the taste. We should consume no more than 2,400 milligrams of sodium daily, the equivalent of one teaspoon—but it includes what has already been added to your food. If you eat processed foods, read their labels carefully; many contain between 25 percent and 45 percent of your daily salt intake in a single serving of that one food—and you still have to eat the rest of your meal! Remove salt and you will watch your bloating go down, foot and ankle swelling subside, and blood pressure plummet. Do this first, then talk to your doctor about reducing or eliminating your medication.

FAQ

Q: I just found out I'm pregnant. I want my baby to grow in a clean environment. Is it safe for me to detox?

A: No. I don't recommend the detox for women who are pregnant or nursing. Because the detox is so powerful, it will dump toxins out of your cells and into your bloodstream, potentially creating a more harmful environment for your baby to grow in than had you not detoxed at all. Nor should you detox while you're breast-feeding, since your baby would then digest very dangerous chemicals in your milk that could undermine his normal development.

Q: I have diabetes and high blood pressure. Is it okay for someone as sick as me to detox?

A: The Martha's Vineyard Diet Detox is not only safe for anyone with an illness, I highly recommend it. High doses of nutrition can repair your body and cause the body to get rid of the toxins that helped make you get sick in the first place. They also replace damaged weak cells with new ones.

thought about, and really follow their inner spirit. In the middle of his detox, one medical doctor decided that it was time to resign from being a physician. After he retired, he began writing poetry and playing the harmonica on Main Street in Martha's Vineyard. One woman I detoxed decided to adopt a baby. A teacher quit school and moved to India to study meditation. When James detoxed for the first time, he decided to get baptized. It was during his detox that he realized that I had to share this information by writing this book. James is an amazing person. Many of my clients are experiencing a spiritual renewal because of him!

Testimonial
THE THREE SISTERS

Name: Loretta Hester
Age: 70
Occupation: retired
Family status: mother of two; grandmother of two
Location: The Woodlands, Texas

I learned about the detox from my son James. I saw how wonderful he looked and felt and I wanted to feel good, too. Middle age had set in and I was starting to gain a lot of weight. I'm not a small person, but I'm short. When I gain weight, I look a little stocky. I had also started feeling very sluggish and tired. James explained the detox and walked me through the steps. At first, it turned me off. I am a sweets eater. I like cake and candy and all the bad stuff. But when he told me the kind of results I could get, I just wanted to do it—I really did! Even though I was nervous and wondered if I would be able to do it, when I set my mind to doing something, I persevere. I knew that I would follow through.

Doing the detox was enjoyable. I didn't feel very hungry, and I lost that sluggish and tired feeling. I lost 21 pounds in 21 days! I looked good, I had a waistline again, I could get back into some of the clothes I really liked, and I could tie my shoes without my stomach getting in the way. And, oh my God, the energy—the absolute energy! I would take walks around the Island that were a couple of miles long and not even get tired. I would walk to church, walk to town, come back, and walk again. My blood pressure also went down. It usually runs about 141/80, but when they took my blood pressure afterwards it was much lower. I thought, "I can't believe this!"

I had just one issue with the detox, and it was the soup—I had a hard time handling the consistency of it. The thickness of it reminded me of pea soup. I came from a family of five girls. I also longed to chew; not chewing was a bit of a challenge.

After I detoxed, my sisters told me, "Loretta, you look great!" I'd say, "You could look like this, too. You'd feel great!" After a couple of years my sister Geri—she's kind of like the leader—said, "We're going to do it together." I said, "That's fine with me," and we did it as a family. That second time I lost 21 pounds in 21 days. James was a wonderful support, and it was great being together. We did a lot of laughing and a lot of sharing and opening up. As she detoxed, one sister who I thought was the Rock of Gibraltar was just crying and letting her feelings out. It was wonderful! I felt so good about myself and good about my sisters. We were so proud of each other!

Name: Geri Trzanowski
Age: 68
Occupation: retired schoolteacher
Residence: Essex Fells, New Jersey
Family status: married; mother of four, grandmother of five

My husband and I entertain and go out to eat a lot. I love to eat and have a big appetite. With me, it's all about food! Now, if you saw me back before I did the detox, I wouldn't have looked overweight to you, but my clothes were uncomfortable and I knew I needed to lose a few pounds. Usually, I would lose weight by cutting down to half portions. But when James told me how much weight I could lose, I said, "That's it, I'm going to try it!" He also explained how healthy it is. That was great, too, but I have to admit that losing weight was the main reason I did it.

Losing weight was great—I lost 20 pounds in 21 days. But my body started feeling so good that I stopped thinking about the weight. I have a lot of arthritis. I used to wake up in the morning wondering, "Which way can I turn over today without it hurting too much?" But even though I walked around the island with my sisters, while I was on the detox I didn't take a pain pill for 21 days! For me this was fabulous! I was amazed to discover that by taking care of my insides I could feel so well. Even today, though I still have pain in my wrist and when it is going to rain I may take an Aleve, I don't need prescription pain pills anymore! Until I detoxed it had never occurred to me that I could get off the pills. I'm thrilled not to have to take them!

For me, detoxing was a great experience. It was difficult but I did it, and my sisters were my support group. Dr. Roni is a dream, and the staff was wonderful. They are really delightful and help you through this. Leaving my family was a huge thing for me to do. I love them and give so much time to them, but I'd never said, "I'm going away for three weeks to take care of myself." I thought this was the greatest gift to give myself. I turned my cell phone off because I wanted the experience to be about me.

These days, I feel so much better than I used to. I'm not saying that I eat properly all the time. And I wouldn't want to detox three weeks again—maybe I'd do it for two weeks. But every so often my husband and I juice and make the soups or we'll have a big lunch and no dinner but a protein shake. And he's always saying, "Let's go up to Martha's Vineyard and do the detox." One day, maybe we will.

Name: Joan Walsh
Age: 66
Occupation: retired public service
Family status: married, mother of three, grandmother of six
Residence: Toms River, New Jersey

I'm the youngest sister. One day, my sister Geri called me and said, "Guess what? Loretta and I are going up to Martha's Vineyard to detox. It would be nice if the three of us could do it together." Well, I'm not a person who goes on vacation. I don't leave my husband, and I thought that detoxes were strictly for alcohol. "What are you talking about?" I asked her. She explained and I told her, "I wish you all the luck in the world but, no, I don't think I want to do that." But Geri is very persuasive, and both my sisters were very excited and talked about how much fun it would be. They got me thinking about how I never go anywhere—with three children and all these grandchildren, I keep very busy. I thought, "Maybe this is a time to take care of me. Let me give it a shot."

So I thought the whole thing would be a nice little getaway, but to be perfectly honest I got roped into going. Later on I learned that she didn't tell me everything. I love to eat. If I'm going to be in Martha's Vineyard, I want to eat. It wasn't until we got there and shopped for vegetables that I realized what all was involved. I started thinking, "Oh, no, this is not going to work." The night before we started, we went out for a very nice dinner. James said, "This is the last one for three weeks.

We're really going to get down to it tomorrow." To be honest with you, I got a little excited. I was about 30 pounds overweight and thought a lot about the idea of cleansing my body. I said to myself, "This isn't going to be all that bad." I was going to go along with everyone else. Whatever they were going to do, I was going to be right there with them.

I did the detox for two weeks. I lost 22 pounds in two weeks and never got hungry. I could not believe I had lost all that weight! I have arthritis and every single day we walked and walked, but I never took a pain pill. My other two sisters went for three weeks, but for me two weeks was enough. In two weeks I had about five colonics. My sister knew about them but she didn't tell me what was going to happen because she knew I wouldn't do them. But to see what is up inside of you—that was unbelievable! I'm not fat but I do have my middle. My middle got smaller after my colonics.

At one point I had a healing crisis. My sisters didn't have one but I had a bad one. For an entire day I was exhausted, completely wiped out. I felt very nauseous and was throwing up. It was like I was getting the flu. I told Dr Roni, "I feel terrible; I can't do this." She explained what was happening. I spent the day in bed. I don't think I've spent an entire day in bed in all my life. It was a very, very bad day. I was angry at my sisters for talking me into doing this. "Please leave me alone"—that's how I felt. Then the next day I woke up and I was fine, as if nothing had happened. In spite of my healing crisis, the detox was a very good experience. It is really a very good program.

4

ALL ABOUT JUICES AND SOUPS

Marsha is a forty-three-year-old medical doctor. She's also a triathlete, competing around the country in high-endurance competitions emphasizing running, biking, and swimming. Before the season begins, she prepares herself by going on a week-long juice fast. Juicing, she says, gives her lots of energy and makes her body quick and limber. She does this at the Inn retreat, where she takes three juices a day. Marsha also claims juicing makes her mind sharp and clear.

Once a year we also host a group of four women bikers. They do a juice fast every year before their twenty-five-mile bike race. Having done this for many years, they know exactly what they are doing. The first time this group of women arrived at our facility, I didn't recognize them as being athletic. I thought they looked tired, stressed out, and pale. Four days later when I saw them again, I literally didn't recognize them. I was shocked by how good these women, who were clearly in their mid-fifties to sixties, looked. Each of them had lost weight, color had returned to their faces, and their personalities were lighter and more fun. Even though I am in this business, even I was amazed.

Juices put oxygen in your body and give you a lot of energy. They're particularly helpful for people who are ill. When people who have been very sick nourish themselves intensively by drinking fresh juice, they can spring back up very quickly. In fact, a review of 4,500 studies conducted around the world found that if people ate at least five servings of fruits and vegetables daily, worldwide cancer rates would drop by more than 20 percent.[1] Other research shows that by eating a variety of fruits and vegetables you can reduce your risk of developing heart disease; high blood pressure; type 2 diabetes; and cancers of the bladder, breast, colon, esophagus, larynx, lungs, mouth, pancreas, pharynx, prostate, ovaries, rectum, and stomach. Though the government recommends that Americans consume at least five servings of fruits and vegetables daily, during the Martha's Vineyard Diet Detox, we're going to consume at least twenty-two servings a day. The vast majority of those will be vegetables, since vegetables both cleanse and feed. It will be easy to eat these extra servings, which we'll drink as fresh live juices and soups.

Maximizing Vegetables' Cleansing Power

Among the best ways to maximize the amount of nutrients we receive from vegetables is to juice them or cook them into delicious veggie soups. While the average person cannot eat a pound of carrots or any other vegetable, they can drink the equivalent amount of juice, and with it consume far more nutrition than they could eat with a knife and fork. You can obtain more nutrients in one eight-ounce glass of fresh vegetable juice than in an entire week's worth of fast-food or take-out meals.

Rather than buying store-bought brands whose enzymes are depleted, we'll make fresh juices so their enzymes are still alive. Enzymes create a spark of life in the body that you can feel as soon as you swallow. Their kick is particularly potent if you're ill or your energy is low. We want to juice our vegetables as soon as possible after they are picked, so more of their enzymes will be alive. Of course, we usually can't know exactly when something was harvested, but we can try to buy produce that's as fresh

---

[1] "Nutrition Can Be Boosted for Low Income Kids with Better After-School Snack Choices, UC Davis Research Confirms," from *Food, Nutrition, and the Prevention of Cancer: A Global Perspective,* a report published by the American Institute for Cancer Research and the World Cancer Research Fund (1997).

as possible; for instance, from a local garden or farmer's market versus flown in from overseas. During the Diet Detox, we will avoid drinking juice that is processed. Remember: processing kills enzymes, making bottled, canned, refrigerated, or frozen options far less effective at cleansing and healing. Most times, refining also means adding preservatives, which are enzyme killers. Juices containing synthetic toxic chemicals usually also contain added salt, which we want to avoid. While some of the vitamins *may* be left in processed juice (the chances of this are greatest with frozen products that don't contain preservatives), without enzymes the body cannot process the juice efficiently, making it more likely to cause digestive difficulties and to turn to fat. Live juice also flushes the acid, resulting in a more alkaline body.

We're going to puree the soups and extract juices we make to achieve the same goal of maximizing nutrients. We'll make our soups and juices fresh, so we get the nutrients without the artificial flavors, colors, and preservatives. You'll find my favorite recipes starting on page 205, but you can stick with recipes you love. While we're detoxing, it's important to avoid putting toxins like salt or seasoning salt or black pepper into them. We'll also avoid eating fruit; sources of protein like meat and beans; dairy products like cheese, milk, and cream; sugar; and wine and alcohol. However, you're free to add as many nonsodium seasonings as you'd like: cayenne pepper, onion, garlic, oregano, basil, cilantro, dill, parsley, curry, cumin, turmeric, thyme, rosemary, paprika, bay leaves, and sage.

Choosing Juices	
Worst	Canned juice
Better	Frozen, preferably with no additives or preservatives; refrigerated, preferably with no additives or preservatives
Best	Fresh, preferably organic

Juicing by Color

When people start juicing, many prefer the flavor of carrots, whose juice is much sweeter than you'd ever expect from eating the vegetable. While juicing a lot of carrots doesn't put you in jeopardy of looking like Bugs Bunny, too much of anything just isn't good for you. And who wants to see their skin turn orange or urine change color (indicators that there's too much of a substance in your system)? It actually happens! The healthiest way to juice is to select vegetables whose colors reflect the entire spectrum from violet to white. For example, you might include vegetables like purple cabbage; violet beets; orange carrots; yellow summer squash; green collards, kale, chard, or broccoli; white cauliflower, white cabbage, garlic, or onions; brown ginger; and garlic. Including vegetables of all these hues is important because each color corresponds to a different set of phytonutrients (natural compounds found in foods that work with vitamins and minerals to promote good health). Including as many colors of vegetables as possible helps ensure we receive the broadest spectrum of healing power available. Research shows that phytonutrients perform the following functions:

- Act as antioxidants
- Stimulate enzymes that detoxify the body
- Stimulate the immune system

The Healing Power of Colors

Color	Vegetable	Phytonutrient
White	Garlic, onions, cauliflower, jicama, parsnips, turnips	Allium, allicin
Yellow/orange	Carrots, summer squash, sweet potatoes	Beta-carotene, bioflavonoid vitamins A and C, potassium
Red	Red cabbage, red onions, red peppers, tomatoes, beets, radishes	Vitamin C, lycopene, and Anthrocyanins
Purple	Purple Belgian endive, eggplant, purple cabbage	Phenolics
Green	Broccoli, celery, cucumbers, greens, and spinach	Indoles, lutein, potassium, vitamin K, zeaxanthin
Brown	Sea vegetables like dried algae, kelp, and kombu	Iodine, vitamin K, folate, magnesium, iron

- Positively affect hormones
- Fight bacteria and viruses

Our goal is to consume as many antioxidants as possible, allowing us to experience their healing effects. While scientists don't yet understand the complete role each of these phytonutrients plays, we *do* know we get sick when we don't get enough of them. While over-the-counter vitamins can be helpful, they do not provide the same type of protection because they do not provide nutrients in the precise combinations that nature intended. Phytochemicals are also contained in fruits, but fruits are foods that feed our cells. During the Martha's Vineyard Diet Detox, our focus is on cleansing and healing, not feeding them. That's why we ingest so many vegetables.

How to Choose a Juicer

Machines that juice fruits and vegetables range from the very inexpensive—those made for "recreational" juicing of, say, the occasional orange when you invite people over for Sunday brunch—to "working" juicers, made for more frequent or productive use. For the Martha's Vineyard Diet Detox, I recommend that you purchase a "working" juicer. There are two different types of "working" juice machines suitable for most detoxers: centrifugal juicers, which first shred the food and then use the centrifugal force that develops as the machine parts spin, to strain it; and masticating juicers that crush vegetables to create the juice and mechanically force its pulp through a strainer. They range in price from $35 to $500. Each type has benefits and disadvantages. Select your juicer based on how much you can afford to spend and how you plan to use it once you complete the detox and begin the Maintenance Program (Chapter 9).

Preparing to Juice

I teach all my clients to create a working kitchen—one that isn't just for show but that helps you look, feel, and be youth-

Finding a Juicer That Is Right for You

Selecting a juicer can be a difficult process. When purchasing a juicer it is important to take into consideration what you need. Do you need a juicer that extracts juice from wheatgrass and spinach or a juicer that makes ice cream? The table below classifies the juicers by type and function to give you an idea of what you may need.

Juicer Pros and Cons

Juicer Type	Pros	Cons
Centrifugal	Requires less preparation; operates at high speed; easy to clean; tends to be less expensive; juices fruits and vegetables.	Not great for soft fruits such as bananas and berries, leafy vegetables, or wheatgrass; causes nutrients to oxidize; creates foam; louder than other juicers.
Masticating (single-gear) or citrus juicer	Extracts more nutrients; preserves more enzymes; processes leafy, green vegetables; quieter than centrifugal machines. Good for making nut butters, pasta, and pureed food. Makes great grapefruit, lemon, and orange juice.	Requires more preparation to cut vegetables into smaller pieces; more force is needed to push vegetables into grinder; produces more pulpy and fibrous juice; tends to be more expensive.
Triturating (twin-gear) juicer	Gives you more fiber, enzymes, vitamins, and trace minerals; excellent for juicing leafy greens, wheatgrass, sprouts, root vegetables like beets and carrots, and most water-dense (nonpulpy) fruits	Juicing takes longer due to the slower machine and two-step juicing process, yielding a higher-quality juice.

Juicer Type	Pros	Cons
Wheatgrass	Used exclusively for extracting the juice from wheatgrass and other leafy greens, as well as some soft fruits like grapes.	Not made for extracting juice from vegetables and most fruits.
Hydraulic press	Very efficient; doesn't waste as much juice.	More expensive (as high as $2,200).

Easy cleanup is one of the most important features to many people who juice, especially if you juice often. You can clean your juicer with hot water and a stiff brush that you obtain at the supermarket. Over time, the juice will stain your machine. Don't worry about this; the purpose of the machine is to help you get healthy, not to look good on your counter. Just follow the manufacturer's directions on how to clean it. Many parts are also dishwasher safe. If easy cleanup is very important to you, you may prefer a centrifugal juicer. If you're ill, need every drop of nutrition you can get, and don't mind longer prep and clean-up times, you may prefer one that masticates. But before you buy any brand, see how much juice it allows you to make before vegetable pulp fills up the clean-up basket. And investigate the length of the warranty, which may run from five to fifteen years.

ful, energetic, and healthy. To me, that means pulling your juicer and other appliances out of the cabinet and placing them front and center among your kitchen implements, like your fork or your butcher knife. Organizing your kitchen saves time and makes your life easier by helping you stay focused. This is particularly important when it comes to juicing, which is a new activity for most people, and one that can eat up time if you're not prepared in advance.

For juicing, if you can afford to buy organic vegetables, by all means you should do it. If not, follow the guidance provided on page 51 and, as you can afford it, include organic versions of some of the vegetables that are known to contain the most contaminants. To keep the cost down, I suggest shopping at food co-ops and farmer's markets, where organic produce is often cheaper than in health-food and gourmet grocery stores. If you can't afford organic at all, don't sweat it. What you are doing now to take care of yourself is better than anything you've ever done. Give yourself a pat on the back!

Before you start juicing, clean your vegetables well. Wash organic produce in warm water only. Conventional produce should be cleaned with a fruit and vegetable cleaner. No matter what kind of produce you buy, use a scrub brush to get into all the nooks and crannies so you don't find yourself drinking dirt.

Cut your vegetables in chunks as large as your juicer can handle right before juicing. Slicing your vegetables right when you use them keeps vital nutrients in the food rather than allowing them to escape into the air. Drink your juice immediately to guarantee that all the nutrients will be intact. Pour it into a glass container and seal the top to prevent oxidation if you are drinking the juice on the go, then store it in a refrigerator and drink it as soon as you can. It's best to drink your juice very fresh, when all the enzymes are active or alive.

FACTOID

A surprising number of people are allergic to what are called "nightshade" vegetables, including eggplant; green, yellow, and red peppers; paprika; potatoes; and tomatoes. Nightshade vegetables can cause inflammation, creating problems like muscle spasms, pain, and stiffness.

Characteristics of Different Juices

Each vegetable (and fruit) contains a unique blend of vitamins, minerals, and phytonutrients. Select from the following commonly juiced vegetables to create your juice blend. You may create combinations based on flavors you enjoy most or on the health benefits you seek. In any case, be sure to include vegetables that reflect the entire spectrum of colors, focusing primarily on green vegetables.

My Favorite Juice Combinations

"Different strokes for different folks," my grandmother would sometimes say. And depending on their tastes, people prefer different types of juice combinations. In the Martha's Vineyard Diet

Juice Name	Vitamins and Minerals	Benefits
Broccoli	Vitamins A, C, E, and K; niacin, folate, potassium, calcium, sulfur, indol-3, carbanol, beta-carotene	A powerful antioxidant and energizer, broccoli juice is too bitter for most people to drink it alone. Try mixing it with carrot juice. Great for cleansing; helps fight cancer and cataracts and performs general healing.
Broccolini (broccoli rabe)	Vitamins C and K	Same as above.
Beet (root and greens)	Iron, calcium, vitamin C, potassium, folate, manganese	Helps to build blood and the immune system as well as fight infection. Great for the liver and gallbladder. Beet juice is one of the most potent juices, so always dilute it with another vegetable like cucumber, celery, and chard.
Carrot	Vitamins A, C, beta-carotene, niacin, folate, B_6, and panthothenic acid	A sweet juice; one of the most powerful antioxidants and detoxifiers. Great for making a juice combination taste better. Helps improve eyesight and acne.
Cabbage	Anthrocyanins, sulfur, beta-carotene, vitamin C	My grandma's favorite vegetable, this potent antioxidant fights cancer, heals stomach ulcers, and improves colon conditions.

Juice Name	Vitamins and Minerals	Benefits
Cauliflower	Vitamins A and C, potassium, folate, calcium, magnesium, phosphorus, indol-3	Cauliflower is hard to juice, but is great for soups. It is a potent cancer-prevention vegetable. Improves digestion and bowel movements, helps to build bone, assists blood formation.
Celery	Sodium; vitamins A, C, and K	Celery's naturally high sodium content helps you replenish natural sodium lost through sweating. So throw your salt shaker in the trash! Excellent for creating glowing skin.
Chard	Vitamin A, C, E, and K; potassium, iron, copper	Prevents digestive tract cancers; has a protective effect on kidneys; helps vision.
Cilantro	Calcium, iron, vitamin C, potassium	Cilantro (Chinese parsley) is used as a spice. It also removes heavy metals, like mercury and aluminum, from the body. It also has antibacterial properties.
Cucumber	Vitamins A, C, and K; manganese, calcium, phosphate, sulfur	Very good for eyesight. Helps to detox kidneys and build the blood.
Fennel	Vitamins C and E, beta-carotene, essential fatty acids, iron, manganese	Good for digestion, relieving gas, and increasing breast milk production.

Juice Name	Vitamins and Minerals	Benefits
Garlic	Allicin	Decreases blood pressure and cholesterol. Acts as an antibacterial and antimicrobial. Helps fight colds and flu and prevent cancer.
Ginger	Vitamin E, selenium, beta-carotene, manganese	Helps relieve nausea and improve the metabolism. Ginger has a strong taste, so don't use too much!
Greens (collard greens, mustard greens, turnip greens)	Iron, calcium indole-3, leonine, potassium, zeaxanthin, vitamins A and C	Greens are very potent antioxidants and blood detoxifiers and are good for the liver. They help relieve constipation and build blood, but it's hard to drink them straight. I mix them with carrot and cucumber juice.
Kale	Vitamins A, C, and K; folate, potassium	Potent antioxidants, detoxifiers, and liver cleaners. Great for improving vision.
Onion	Lycopene, anthrocyanins, allium, allicin, selenium, manganese, potassium, phosphate, vitamin C, folate	Onion is a potent blood purifier. It assists with skin and wound healing.
Parsnip	Vitamins C and K, manganese, folate, potassium	A great antioxidant and detoxifier.
Peppers (green)	Niacin, folate, potassium, iron, niacin, selenium, vitamins A and C	Green peppers are a great seasoning and help to break down protein. They are nightshade foods so should be avoided during the detox.

Juice Name	Vitamins and Minerals	Benefits
Radish	Folic acid, calcium, potassium, and dietary fiber	Helps to clean the blood and detoxify the body.
Spinach	Vitamin A, C, and K; folate, potassium, phosphate, selenium, iron	Good for blood formation and fighting anemia, spinach makes you stronger and is a potent detoxifier.
Sweet potato	Vitamins C and B_6, niacin, pantothenic acid, folate, potassium, phosphate, magnesium, selenium	Sweet and healthy enough to help the liver to repair. It gives you energy and strength, which makes it popular among athletes.
Tomato	Lycopene, vitamins B_6 and C, anthrocyanins	Fights prostate cancer
Turnip	Vitamin C, manganese, copper, potassium	Contains very potent antioxidants, detoxifies the liver, and helps to keep bones healthy.

SOURCES: Vitamin and Mineral Chart by George Carter and Jen Curry; Dr. Decuypere's Nutrient Chart; HealthAlternatives2000.com.

Detox, we juice for nutrition more than for flavor. You may have to get used to the taste of the different vegetable juices. But if we can grow to enjoy the acidic tastes of beer and hard liquor, we can certainly swig eight ounces of something healthy if that's what we need to do to get it past our tongue. Here are some of my favorite juice combinations to treat different health conditions:

- Arthritis: bean sprout, carrot, cucumber, fennel, kale, parsnip, turnip (wheatgrass alone)
- Cancer: broccoli, kale, carrot, beet, beet greens
- Fluid retention: bean sprout, cucumber, fenugreek sprout, watercress
- Heart disease: spinach, broccoli, beets, garlic

- High cholesterol: turnips, dandelion, carrot, spinach, parsley, ginger root
- Impotence: kale, alfalfa sprouts, lambs quarter (wheatgrass alone)
- Liver problems: beets, dandelion greens, parsnips, endive, spinach
- Menopause: Swiss chard, watercress, bean sprouts, beet greens
- Prostate problems: asparagus, parsley, tomatoes, watercress
- Ulcers: cabbage, kale, carrot, parsnips (wheatgrass alone)

I like these juices because of their flavorful or refreshing taste:

- 5 carrots, 4 collard leaves, 2 parsley sprigs, ¼ beet
- 4 spinach leaves, 4 turnip leaves, 4 kale leaves, 5 carrots, ¼ clove garlic
- 4 broccoli florets, ½ cucumber, 3 carrots, ¼ inch of ginger
- 1 cucumber, 1 beet, 3 beet leaves, 3 carrots, ¼ clove garlic
- 1 cup green beans, 5 leaves of spinach, 5 carrots

Hint . . .

- Juice if you're really thirsty.
- Juice if you need salt or are craving salt.
- Juice if you need energy.

Making Fresh Soups

Another way of obtaining maximum nutrition in minimum doses is by eating specially prepared soups. To keep things simple, feel free to make a variation of a soup you're familiar with. For instance, you can take one of your favorite winter soups and remove any white flour, white rice, sweetener, milk/cream, meat, butter, and salt from the recipe. Of course, the soup will taste differently than you are used to, but remember your focus here is to nourish yourself in a way that allows you to lose weight, not in satisfying a culinary critic. That said, there's no need to suffer through a lousy-tasting meal. Feel free to pump up the other flavors in the soup—adding more garlic, onions, cilantro, or parsley, for instance—to satiate your taste buds. You can be creative and combine your own ingredients and seasonings. The combinations are endless. For instance, if you want an Italian-inspired soup, you may choose to combine broccoli, carrots, cauliflower, onions, yellow squash, and zucchini, topping them off with basil, oregano, parsley, and rosemary. (Depending on your body chemistry, you may or may not want to include potatoes, tomatoes, or other nightshade vegetables.) If you prefer a sweeter soup, you may want to combine carrots, onions, and sweet potatoes with a little cinnamon and nutmeg and vanilla extract. You can use any herbs you like for flavor. Here are some of my favorite combinations. You don't need to worry about proportions; season to taste instead.

- Celery, collard greens, green beans, onion, and sweet potato, seasoned with cayenne pepper, cumin, curry, garlic (chopped), ginger (chopped)
- Carrots, cauliflower, green beans, and kale, seasoned with bay leaves, Cajun seasoning (salt-free version), cilantro, garlic powder, parsley
- Broccoli, celery, chard, kale, onions, scallions, and spinach, seasoned with cayenne pepper, garlic, salt-free seasoning
- Carrots, cauliflower, green beans, onions, and spinach, seasoned with garlic and vegetable seasoning (salt-free version)

Note: Carrots, beets, and sweet potatoes will make your soup sweeter, but the goal is to keep your soup as green as possible.

Making the soup is easy. Place 2 cups of cut-up vegetables in a large pot (or you can cook overnight in a crock pot). Add 4 cups of water. Cook until softened (about 10 to 20 minutes, depending on what vegetables you choose). Add herbs and spices to taste. If you feel like Italian, add basil, bay leaf, oregano, rosemary leaves, or sage. Enjoy Cajun? Add cayenne pepper, paprika, oregano,

How to Cheat and Get Away With It

There are days during which even the most devoted detoxer feels the overwhelming urge to eat. On those days, I strongly encourage you to cheat. But instead of pigging out on a bag of Oreos, jump off of the plan in a way that supports your weight loss. The best way is by drinking what I call "free soup" (many of you know it as "pot liquor"). Free soup is broth designed to provide you with some minerals and fluids along with a strong taste that will take the edge off. The calories you ingest in free soup are offset by the number of calories your body uses in the process of digesting the soup. It contains low-calorie, leafy vegetables prepared with strong, tasty spices. Here's how to make it:

In a large pot, place 2 cups of cut-up vegetables such as celery, cilantro, collard greens, cucumbers, garlic, kale, onions, spinach, watercress. (*Note:* The soup must include at least one dark green vegetable.) Add 4 cups of water, followed by your favorite spices, such as cayenne, cumin, curry, paprika, turmeric, or vegetable seasoning without salt. Simmer until vegetables are softened, about 30 to 60 minutes or use a Crock-Pot to simmer all day. Spoon one cup of vegetables into a blender and blend until liquid. Using a slotted spoon, scoop out the rest of the vegetables and discard. Pour the blended vegetables back into the soup broth in the pot. Drink up all day, knowing that you're taking the edge off your hunger without increasing stress on your digestive system. This is a time when it is not about calories.

onion, and garlic. My favorite is Indian, so I add curry, cumin, coriander, cinnamon, and turmeric to a soup made with broccoli, carrots, sweet potato, and green beans. Or check out the recipes on pages 205–208. For an energy boost, add 1 teaspoon of the sea vegetables kelp or dulse, which add a wide variety of minerals. Remove the vegetables from the pot and puree in a blender. Set the broth aside to drink during the day.

5

SUPPLEMENTS YOU'LL NEED DURING THE DETOX

Peter (name changed), a forty-three-year-old married father of three, was proud of being a "meat and potatoes" man. "I don't do vegetables," he informed me on the day we started working together.

"You won't eat one vegetable?" I asked.

"Never!" he answered. "I will never do vegetables."

I wondered if maybe his parents pushed him too much as a child so he decided never to eat another veggie in life.

Unbeknownst to Peter, his unwillingness to eat green foods was taking its toll on his body. He had a beer belly and needed to lose about 50 pounds. He did not look his age at all—he had so many wrinkles I thought he was at least fifteen to twenty years older. I could tell his body was very acidic.

Unfortunately, Peter's situation is not that unusual. Most Americans do not get enough vegetables, and if it weren't for french fries, many would eat hardly any. Yet vegetables are vital to the body's well-being. They are the only food group that cleanses as well as feeds our cells. But even though the government recommends that we eat between five and nine servings of vegetables and fruits each day, the average American eats only one!

Compounding matters, when we do eat vegetables, they usually don't have enough nutrients in them—and let's not forget that they contain toxic chemicals! That's why it is important to take nutritional supplements. Now, I'm not just talking about any old supplement—I don't mean the chemically synthetic vitamins you buy at the grocery store. I'm talking about a high-density, powdered nutritional supplement that's actually made from fruits and vegetables. These nutrient-dense products give you several days' worth of nutrition in a single eight-ounce glass—more than you could eat in one sitting. Down one drink, and you've consumed enough fruits and vegetables for the entire day. While I don't suggest that anyone use them to replace fruits and vegetables entirely, they're ideal for people like Peter—as well as everyday folks who would eat more veggies if they had the time. While you're on the Martha's Vineyard Diet Detox, you will take them several times daily along with other supplements to support your body's cleanse.

Green Drinks

One of the most important high-density supplements I include in the Martha's Vineyard Diet Detox is known as a "green drink," which is usually derived from green vegetables. Before growing into the mature grains that land in our breakfast bowls and on our dinner tables, cereals like wheat, barley, and rye begin their life cycle as grasses. While they're young, tender, and grassy, these grains are particularly high in nutrition. Their nutrients are densely concentrated—much more so than in the full-grown plant. These grasses (and other greens) feed many of the biggest animals on the planet—cows, elephants, horses, oxen, and buffalo, for example. The phrases "as strong as an ox" and "as strong as a horse" originate in the power packed in these grasses, which help the body oxygenate the cells. The result? Green drinks clean your system, give you energy, and make your body more alkaline. Once you start taking them, your hair and skin will look wonderful! Because they exist in liquid form, the nutrients within them reach your cells very quickly. Many people who drink them say they experience a type of high.

Wheatgrass, in particular, gives the body a lot of get-up-and-go. You may be familiar with it already since it's served frequently at juice bars. Wheatgrass is perhaps the most powerful cleansing, nourishing, and energizing food—it's served in tiny "shot" glasses. Even then, not everyone can handle it. It gives some people so much energy, they can't drink it after mid-afternoon or they'll lie awake well into the night. In fact, it is such a strong cleaner that some people can't tolerate it until they detoxify. If their body is very toxic, wheatgrass may cleanse their body so quickly it will cause them to projectile vomit! (This is a healing crisis).

Now, please bear with me briefly while I explain some of the science behind green grasses. They contain lots of chlorophyll, the green pigment that absorbs light energy from the sun. Chlorophyll transforms that solar energy into adenosine triphosphate (ATP), a molecule that stores energy and transports it between the cells. In photosynthesis, the process plants use to turn sunlight into food, chlorophyll plays a major role. So when you consume the grasses of these grains and other green foods, you're actually eating sunrays that have been transformed into food. No other foods provide you with more energy!

The green drink I've included in the Martha's Vineyard Diet Detox is a high-density nutrient powder primarily composed of grasses like the ones mentioned above. It also contains vegetables like broccoli, greens, and kale; spirulina; and blue-green algae that is one of the most nutrient-dense plants on Earth. These grasses, vegetables, and fruits are harvested at their peak and then are dried and lightly processed into powders. This high-tech process preserves most of their vitamins, minerals, nutrients, phytochemicals, and enzymes but leaves the fiber behind. You just mix a scoop of green supplement with water, which I prefer, or juice. Most provide as much nutrition in a single eight-ounce glass as eight to ten servings of vegetables. While salads and steamed vegetables don't always fit into your purse, green drinks are road ready. You can buy packets of powder and carry them with you, scoop powder into a Ziploc bag, or pour it into your water bottle, shake it, and drink whenever you're ready!

Green drinks have been around for a long time, so the technology has improved considerably. If you tried them back in the early days, you may have been turned off by their taste, since the first-generation drinks were composed only of grasses, vegetables, and algae. They tasted, well . . . very green! Fortunately, times have changed. Today, many contain apples, bananas, berries, carrots, and other sweeter fruits and vegetables. They actually taste good. Some green drinks contain only spirulina or barley. You don't want that type for the Martha's Vineyard Diet Detox; you will need a broader spectrum of nutrients. Instead, choose one with as many different green grasses and vegetables in it as you can find. Ideally, the ingredients will be organic, with no added sugars, salt, or preservatives. During your detox, you'll consume a green drink at least twice a day.

I have to admit that getting Peter to consume a green drink was a challenge. (I gave up on the vegetables early on and thought I'd try stealth green drinks instead.) It took me several days to figure out how to do it, but in a few days I was able to sneak one into Peter's regimen without his knowledge. Many of the drinks taste so good I knew the trick was to disguise the drink's color so that it didn't look green. I used one of the old-style plastic water bottles with an opaque plastic top and a straw.

"Do you know what you drank?" I asked him. "Five servings of fruits and vegetables!"

Peter couldn't believe it. As he continued with the program, not only did he detox and shed 21 pounds, he lost years off his face (www.mvdietdetox.com).

Antioxidant Berry Drinks

Even though people seem to enjoy the flavor of fruits a lot more than they like veggies, Americans don't eat enough of them. And when we do eat fruit, we typically consume the usual apple, orange, or banana, rather than the variety our body truly needs. I tell my clients that one trick I use that helps me consume more fruits is squeezing fresh lemon or lime juice into my water. On hot summer days when I'm not detoxing, I enjoy a salad containing mangos, papaya, pineapple, and watermelon. But even though I eat enough fruit, I know it no longer packs the potency that it should. In 1955, one orange contained approximately 50 mg of vitamin C; today, it only contains about 5 mg. The same is true with peaches, another of my favorites. As much as I love them, I can't eat the twenty-five I'd now have to eat to obtain a full day's supply of vitamin C.

So since an apple a day no longer keeps the doctor away, it's important to take an antioxidant supplement. Like green drinks, these supplements provide high doses of phytonutrients, in particular, disease-fighting antioxidants, which are found mostly in fruits, particularly berries. Many fruits—blueberries, pomegranates, grapes, blackberries, prunes (dried plums), and raspberries among them—are "superfoods," foods that scientists have discovered pack tremendous amounts of antioxidants and, therefore, do more than their share of nourishing, healing, and preventing. Antioxidant drinks are powerful and particularly helpful for people whose bodies and joints are inflamed and those who are full of toxins. Premenopausal women find that they help their bodies retain less fluid.

While you're on the Martha's Vineyard Diet Detox, you'll consume one antioxidant berry drink daily. Each glass provides the nutritional equivalent of six to eight servings of fruit, mostly berries. Choose one containing as many different kinds of berries in it as possible. I particularly like the exotic taste of those made with acai berry, wolfberry, goji berry, and noni. Your antioxidant supplement should also have a high oxygen radical absorbance capacity (ORAC) value. ORAC measures the potency of the antioxidants in the drink. The U.S. Food and Drug Administration (FDA) recommends that we get 7,000 ORAC units daily, the equivalent of five to ten fruits and vegetables. Your antioxidant berry drink should also contain no added sugar, salt, or preservatives. Your green drinks should have a variety of berries, not just one kind (www.mvdietdetox.com).

Digestive Enzymes

When we eat the standard American diet, we end up enzyme deficient. When we're short on digestive enzymes—either because there are inadequate amounts in our food or because our body no longer produces enough of its own—after we eat we feel it in the form of abdominal pain, bloating, constipation, diarrhea, gas, nausea, and even vomiting. Sometimes we experience these and other symptoms—say, itching or a rash—because we have food allergies we're unaware of, allergies that enzymes naturally help treat. Thank goodness, we can buy digestive enzymes at the health-food store that are similar to the ones the body manufactures in our stomach. By taking supplements containing protease, amylase, lipase, and cellulase, we can assist and speed up digestion and minimize the effects of food allergens. I like to think of these enzymes as being a lot like the old video game character "Pac Man" since they engulf and "eat" foreign substances as they clean the digestive tract. After taking them you will experience less bloating almost immediately. You'll also have more energy after your meals. During the Diet Detox, you will take digestive enzymes before drinking your vegetable juice and soup. When your detox is over, I suggest staying on them since our food supply lacks them (www.mvdietdetox.com).

Aloe Vera

Aloe vera is a greenish-grey plant with sharp, spiky, succulent leaves. Though native to Africa, the plant is hardy and its medicinal uses so popular that it is now found around the world. Most Americans are aware of aloe's anti-inflammatory effect and use it to treat minor cuts, burns, and skin rashes. I used to keep several plants on my kitchen windowsill for precisely that purpose. Aloe also moisturizes, making it a popular ingredient in beauty products for hair and skin. While you're on the Martha's Vineyard Diet Detox, you will take aloe vera as a nutritional supplement. Taken internally, aloe supplies antiaging antioxidants; helps to restore pH balance and repair cellular health; has a mild laxative effect, making it easier to move your bowels; and improves colon health. In fact, research suggests it is very therapeutic in chronic colon conditions like colitis (www.mvdietdetox.com).

Herbal Cleansing Formula

Herbs work in a synergistic way to encourage organs to flush harmful toxins and elements out of the body. They flush the elimination organs, such as the kidney, liver, and colon, by cleansing their insides. Some herbs, such as cayenne pepper and ginger, stimulate the body, making you feel increased energy; others have a cleansing effect. In combination, the herbs cleanse, repair, or build specific organs, improving the digestive system. For example, herbs can help clear mucus off the colon walls, repair inflammation in the colon, clean out the kidneys to help them keep our system more alkaline, and normalize liver function to keep our hormones balanced. In essence, herbs can increase our metabolic rate and improve our overall health. These are some of the most effective: dandelion root, alfalfa leaf, black cohosh, burdock root, cascara sagrada, psyllium seed husk, beet fiber, oat bran, apple pectin, rice fiber, fennel seed, and slippery elm bark.

Protein Drink

If you are among the few detoxers who want to cleanse their body without losing weight, you should consume one or two protein drinks daily. Look for a brand made from soy, eggs, and/or whey (the liquid remaining after milk has been curdled and strained), that contains ingredients you're not allergic to, all nine essential amino acids, and more protein than carbohydrates. While you're on your detox, mix your drink with water or soy, rice, or almond milk rather than cow's milk, depending on the product directions. For additional flavor, add natural extracts like vanilla, cinnamon, almond, or banana (www.mvdietdetox.com).

Testimonial
ROSALIE FOREST

Age: 40
Occupation: software engineer and aspiring actress
Location: Catonsville, Maryland

Back when I started the Martha's Vineyard Diet Detox, I was feeling really bad about myself. To tell you the truth, I was feeling miserable, ashamed, and depressed. Over the years I had crept up from a size 9/10 to a 12, then to a 14, and even that had started feeling tight. I knew it was only a matter of time before I was wearing a size 16. I couldn't let that happen—I have a daughter who needs her mother to be healthy enough to take care of her! All told, I had gained about 40 pounds. It hurt to look in the mirror, and when I would see myself in photos, I would ask, "Who is that?"

In addition to being hard to deal with emotionally, those 40 pounds were taking a physical toll. I suffered from severe migraines. I always felt tired and had become unable to engage in a lot of the physical activities I used to enjoy. My heart felt like I was about to have a heart attack—I felt like I was literally about to expire. I actually felt so poorly that I went to my doctor and requested a complete physical. When the lab tests returned, my physician surprised me by saying, "I have bad news . . . I can't find *anything* wrong with you." All of my lab tests had come back perfect: my heart was strong, my blood was fine, and there were no signs of any medical conditions! Together, we reached the conclusion that the reason I was feeling so bad had to be the excess weight.

Feeling unhappy and ashamed of myself was draining me emotionally, mentally, and now physically. I knew I had to do something, but what? I had tried other weight-loss programs. Only one worked, and the results were short term. As soon as I stopped the program, I gained back all of the weight plus some. So when I read in *Sister to Sister* magazine about the success its publishers Lorenzo and Jamie Foster Brown had experienced on the Martha's Vineyard Diet Detox, I was extremely excited. Could I really lose 21 pounds in 21 days? That spring while getting spa treatments on a cruise, I had learned about toxins, the effect they have on the body, and how they contribute to weight gain. Here was an opportunity to detox and lose weight, too? Sign me up, I thought. What did I have to lose but shame, misery, and unwanted weight? I was eager to see the results!

So I reached out to Dr. Roni, knowing I couldn't travel to Martha's Vineyard but hoping that there was another alternative. She explained that I could detox at home using her online program (www.mvdiet detox.com). My primary goal was to lose the weight—I eventually wanted to lose 30 pounds. I also wanted to eliminate toxins. I hoped that detoxing would help me look and feel better and gain a new outlook on life. I wanted to look like the "me" that I was used to seeing, rather than this "other person" who looked back at me in the mirror. I desperately wanted not to feel miserable and ashamed of myself.

Doing the detox required that I make a significant lifestyle change that I was not used to. To go from eating and drinking anything I wanted to literally drinking vegetable juices, broths, and minerals and eating green mushy stuff was truly a hard adjustment. It seemed like I saw and smelled food more than I ever had before. It was hard having to cook for my daughter and take her out to eat, but not being able to eat the way I was used to. But once I began to see the results, it was very easy to stick with it. I was surprised to see how quickly I lost weight—I averaged about one pound a day. It was amazing to get on the scale and just see the weight melting away. Before I knew it, my clothes were falling off and everyone was asking me if I had lost weight. My eyes were clearer, and the dry and dull skin I had suffered all my life began to look shiny and healthy. My hair even looked great. All this was noticeable very quickly!

By the end of the 21-day detox, I had lost 36.5 pounds! It wasn't until then that I learned I had been the first person to try her at-home approach. Subsequently, I have done the 7-day maintenance program every three months. I have maintained a 25- to 28-pound weight loss. I can't tell you how much I love having more energy and self-esteem and being a happier, healthier me. My heart feels stronger and less stressed, and I don't get migraines as frequently. When I do get one, I believe it's my body telling me it's time to detox again! I am no longer ashamed to look at myself in the mirror or photographs.

It feels great to wear a bikini and get an admiring stare instead of a frown! I have been amazed by how much kinder people are when you are smaller compared to how mean they can be when you're overweight. Now that I have more energy, I exercise more and am able to engage in physical activities I couldn't or didn't want to before. And with this kind of success under my belt, these days it's easy for me to detox, in spite of all the temptations around me. I never thought it would be so easy to "just say no" to food.

6

UNDERSTANDING ELIMINATION THERAPY

While I was still a full-time nurse, another nurse told me the story of a mentally challenged man who had come to the emergency room because he was feeling extremely sick. His abdomen was as distended as that of a woman who was five months pregnant. It turns out he was very constipated. Once the staff discovered that he was literally full of you know what, they didn't feeling like being bothered. So rather than give him an enema to help clean out his colon and talking to him about improving his diet to find out why he became so constipated in the first place, they just gave him some laxatives and sent him on his way. Well, I don't know if he took the laxatives or not, but he must have kept on eating the same foods that had put his digestive system in gridlock. He still couldn't poop. Tragically, before long, he died of toxemia—too many toxins in the blood.

While this is an extreme example of someone whose eliminatory system was not operating properly, I see many patients who experience problems of one kind or another with moving their bowels. I have talked to many people who have not eliminated their bowels in two weeks, not realizing that some of the symptoms they're experiencing—signs such as mood swings, depression, headaches, brain fog, joint pain, and fatigue—are simply due to the fact that they have too many toxins in their body that can't get out.

Because the Martha's Vineyard Diet Detox causes the cells to scrub themselves so rapidly, it is exceedingly important that we get the noxious substances out of our body before they build up in our bloodstream and make us feel "off" or actually become sick. I want you to take a proactive approach that will help you remove toxins pronto. After the detox, I strongly suggest that you incorporate these techniques into your self-care regimen to help you take better care of yourself and keep your system clean.

The Process of Elimination

The human digestive tract is essentially a thirty-foot tube that begins at our mouth and ends at our anus. While we think of digestion as occurring in our stomach, it actually begins before food hits our mouth. Our sense of smell tells the body to secrete extra saliva. Our saliva chemically breaks down our food, enhancing the chewing process. If you chew thoroughly, the food is reduced to mush that is ready to be digested by the stomach. If you don't— and most Americans don't—some of the work that was supposed to have been done in the mouth now must take place in the stomach, causing us to experience gas, bloating, and indigestion. So it's important to masticate very well—100 chews per bite of food.

After we swallow, our food travels down our esophagus to our stomach, which liquefies and begins to digest it. Our stomach then sends the partially digested food to our small intestine, where the pancreas, gallbladder, kidneys, and liver chip in and metabolize this substance into molecules—for instance, starch is transformed into simple sugars, protein into amino acids, fats are broken down so that they dissolve in water—that are small enough to pass through the wall of the small intestine. Once these nutrients, which are now punier than a pinpoint, pass through the intestinal wall, they enter the bloodstream, which carries them to every cell. While that's going on, the waste left over from the food you ate continues down the digestive tract, traveling out of the small intestine into the large intestine or colon, a squiggly tube about five feet long. After the cells eat, they eliminate waste, which travels through microscopic pathways that meet back up with the colon, which essentially throws out the entire body's trash each time you move your bowels.

While it's pretty easy to understand how food moves from your stomach to your small intestine and into your colon as waste, the process by which cells empty the trash is much more mysterious. Our eliminatory system consists of an intricate labyrinth of pathways running all throughout the body. The large intestine (colon), the superhighway on which waste travels on its way out of the body, is the most obvious. But before waste reaches this freeway, trash travels along invisible byways and through our bloodstream by way of our veins and arteries that ultimately flow to our colon. If we think of the colon as the body's eliminatory "superhighway," then the smaller pathways are similar to the smaller traffic arteries that crisscross any city. The "driveways" that serve each cell dump trash into the smaller arteries and veins—side streets, if you will. These, in turn, intersect with main streets, then major arteries, on-ramps, highways, and, ultimately, our superhighway—the colon.

In a well-functioning body, the cells empty their trash and trash-hauling *phagocytes* carry it away through this waste-elimination system, eating up as many noxious substances as possible along the way. Ultimately, these toxins reach the colon, where they ride the wavelike motions of peristalsis and exit the body. But in a body whose toxic burden is high, the phagocytes as well as other cleansing cells and organs can become saturated and overwhelmed. Just as a city's transportation system gets crowded and experiences choke points and accidents that slow its flow, its byways slow down and exit routes get congested. At this point symptoms become noticeable. Classic signs of a toxic body include being overweight, fatigue, foggy thinking, body odor, achy joints, swelling, and inflammation. When conditions get really bad, as the constipated man I mentioned experienced, the entire body can go into gridlock as bad as New York on Thanksgiving weekend. The brain behaves similarly to an "eye in the sky" traffic helicopter, figuring out where all of the "choke points" are and telling the body to automatically seek out alternate routes for the toxins to travel. But in some people's bodies, even the back streets get jammed. Sometimes conditions get so bad that the cells have tremendous difficulty in throwing out their trash. Of course, by the time this happens the person is usually very sick.

Constipation is both a common symptom and cause of a toxic body. Ideally, after you eat, the waste from that meal should push the trash from earlier meals down the pipeline, causing you to have a bowel movement. In fact, that's my rule of thumb: when food enters the top of the large intestine, feces should come out the bottom. In countries where people eat healthy whole foods that still contain their vital nutrients and have few artificial ingredients, people have more than one bowel movement a day. This is ideal. But the standard American diet slows our digestive system, even clogs it, making us backed up. In this society I think that if you have three bowel movements a day (one following your three meals) you're doing exceptionally; two are good; one is the minimum that will support good health. Going less often means you're constipated. Now, we all may experience constipation on occasion—because we eat denatured food or are traveling, for instance. But chronic constipation means that your body is circulating toxins looking for a way to get them out or store them in some out-of-the-way place—and that sets you up to get sick.

I'll tell you up front that my perspective conflicts with that of the American Gastrological Association (AGA), the professional organization representing doctors who specialize in gastrointestinal tract diseases. The AGA states that the "normal frequency" of bowel movements "varies widely, from three bowel movements a day to three a week." A person is constipated, they say, "if more than three days pass between bowel movements or if there is difficulty or pain when passing a hardened stool."

However, I'm less concerned with what is so-called "normal" and more concerned with what's healthy. More than that, I like my advice to make sense. Does theirs? You decide. Consider what would happen if on several consecutive 98.6-degree days—the temperature of the human body—you decided not to take out the trash. Now I'm not talking about paper trash, I'm talking about food scraps. It wouldn't take long for the fruits, vegetables, starches, and grains to ferment and decompose, creating a gas that would "light up" your house. The fatty products like mayonnaise or bacon grease would turn rancid. It may take a couple of days, but you'd smell them, too. And the meat would begin to rot, emitting that all-too-familiar, way-past-its-sale-date odor and spawning maggots, which would be crawling all over it. This is exactly what happens when waste sits in your body—it breaks down, ferments, turns rancid, smells, rots, and hatches parasites. If you're not having at least one bowel movement daily, I can guarantee you're having some of these problems:

- Abdominal bloating and gas—happens when decaying foods ferment.
- Acid reflux—in some cases heartburn happens because there's not enough room for the food to go down, so it tries to come back up.
- Stomach upset and nausea—just the idea of fermenting, rancid, and rotting ingredients mixing it up in your belly probably turns your stomach now.
- Stomachaches—doesn't it make sense that your digestive organs would hurt if they had to expand to accommodate gas and waste?
- Body odor—the reason that some people have a wicked body odor is because their digestive system is so backed up that the odor is literally excreted through their pores.
- Excess abdominal weight—many people's abdomens are literally stuffed full of feces.

Many of these problems originate in the colon, the five to six feet of the digestive pipeline that precede the final six inches, or *rectum*. A healthy colon consists of pink, flexible, and supple tissue about the texture and consistency of your skin. It's lined with many nooks and crannies. Like skin, it has microscopic pores in it that allow water and electrolytes, such as sodium, along with any nutrients the small intestine might have missed, to flow through the colon's walls and into the bloodstream. The colon is very sensitive because it is made up of many types of tissues, including muscle. When it feels waste enter at the top, the muscles begin to pulsate and contract, propelling the waste matter through the colon and into the rectum, a process known as peristalsis. But many factors interfere with this process, including:

- Toxins
- Synthetic and artificial ingredients in the waste the body was unable to digest
- Insufficient fiber
- Missing essential fatty acids (EFAs)
- Low levels of digestive flora, also known as "good bacteria," or enzymes
- Too many bad bacteria
- Not enough enzymes to assist with digestion

When the body experiences these types of conditions, waste and synthetic substances build up along the inside of the colon, creating a thick, black, and slimy sludge. Over time, this fecal matter hardens and develops the consistency of a rubber tire. Because the colon's inner walls are now covered with this rubbery stuff, they can't feel the arriving waste matter and don't engage in peristalsis as effectively. When the colon behaves sluggishly, feces linger longer. Not surprisingly, this creates even more slime. As the sludge thickens, the passageway through the colon narrows, just as happens with your household pipes when they clog with grease and debris. As this happens, the shape of our stool changes. Healthy feces are medium brown, roughly two feet long, the diameter of a half dollar, smell but do not have a noxious odor, and float on the top of the water. Unhealthy stools are slender or small—think: pencil-thin, rock or pebble sized—sink to the bottom of the toilet, and "light up" the bathroom and maybe several surrounding rooms. If your bowel movements display any of these characteristics, something is obstructing or interfering with its normal behavior and you need to take action. Most of the time the culprit is impacted waste. *Many people have between ten and twenty-five pounds of toxic fecoid matter just sitting in their colon!* I didn't believe my colon therapist back when I was sick and she quoted me that statistic. But once I started getting colonics, I lost weight like crazy! Sometimes issues more significant than sludge slow the elimination system. Health issues whose causes range from the easy-to-solve—not consuming enough fiber or water, for example—to more onerous, like having a tumor, can interfere with bowel movements. These types of problems can cause bleeding and turn stools black, create mucus in the stools, or cause a sense of fullness that exists even on an empty stomach. Very light-colored stools—usually gray or almond-colored—also signal health problems. If you experience any of the above, there is reason for concern, so contact your doctor immediately.

Whether you have two pounds or twenty pounds of sludge coating your colon, if it is stuck there decaying and putrefying, it is creating gas and causing bloating and other digestive problems. Because the colon's walls are semipermeable, trapped toxins pass back into the bloodstream, where they circulate around the body, making us look and feel sick and tired. The body attempts to take toxins out of circulation by storing them as fat. Sometimes, sludge coating the colon wall blocks an on-ramp connecting that organ to one of the highways carrying in waste from another part of the body. Not surprisingly, traffic on that byway then backs up, and toxins from the body part it serves can't download into the colon quickly enough. If the backup is bad enough, the trash will overflow into a waterway known as the lymphatic system, congesting cellular tissues along its route. Disease results in the far-off region that's unable to cleanse itself. That's why many experts in complementary and alternative medicine believe that disease begins in the colon.

Since our environment and food supply expose us to an incredible number of synthetic chemicals that the body does not know how to process, I strongly believe that we need assistance in keeping our colons clean. This is especially true if you are among the many Americans who do not move your bowels at least once daily. Because man-made chemicals cannot be processed by the organs, the other body systems that help us eliminate toxins—the liver, kidneys, lymphatic system, gallbladder, and skin—need assistance with cleansing as well.

The Liver

Weighing in at over three pounds and located on the right side of the abdomen beneath the diaphragm, the liver is the body's largest glandular organ. The liver filters more toxins out of your system than any other organ and engages in over a hundred vital body functions. For one, it is a fat-burning machine. Using a soap-powder-like cleanser called bile that is produced in the gallbladder, the liver breaks fat down into a liquid that's able to travel through the wall of the small intestine and into the bloodstream. When the body is very toxic, the liver works inefficiently, becoming congested and less effective in breaking down fats. As a result, we are unable to lose weight efficiently, making weight loss harder. Another vital role the liver plays is in maintaining blood concentrations of glucose by storing or releasing glucose as needed. Carbohydrates are stored as glycogen in the liver and are released as energy between meals or when the body's energy demands are high. In this way, the liver helps to regulate the blood sugar level and to prevent a condition called hypoglycemia (low blood sugar). This enables us to keep an even level of energy throughout the day. Without this balance, we would need to eat constantly to keep up our energy.

The liver already has a very difficult job. But its work is made even harder if your digestive system isn't working well. If you are constipated, for instance, there may not be enough digestive enzymes or stomach acid to completely digest our food. The standard American diet causes most people to have one or more of these problems, putting additional stress on the liver. A sluggish liver burns fat inefficiently and can contribute to hormonal imbalances, memory problems, fatigue, depression, bloating, and other symptoms. When the herbalist told me that I had to eat baby food, I remember that the whites of my eyes were yellowish, indicating liver malfunction. If your liver functions poorly, it affects your entire health.

The Kidneys

A poorly functioning colon also affects the kidneys. Our kidneys maintain the harmony of the body's internal environment. Among the processes they manage are removing waste products generated by the metabolic process, drugs, toxins, and other unneeded sub-stances that have been absorbed by the digestive tract; releasing hormones that help the body produce red blood cells, regulate blood pressure, and maintain our bones; keeping the blood at the slightly alkaline pH of 7.35 to 7.45; and helping maintain the volume and concentration of urine. How much people urinate can vary from person to person, as well as from day to day. Urine volume can be as little as one cup per day—such a person would be very toxic—to as much as twenty-four cups! Drinking adequate amounts of water helps the kidneys do a better job of flushing out your system.

The Lymphatic System

The lymphatic system is a microscopic detoxifying highway run-ning immediately beneath the skin's surface. It connects to every one of the trillion cells in your body, and its job is to collect cel-lular waste and debris, fat, bacteria, viruses, toxins, and water, and return them back to the bloodstream, where they are routed to the eliminatory organs for disposal. When you're toxic, your lymphatic system works tremendously hard. When you detox it moves a tre-mendous amount of fat and toxins being flushed out of the cells. Unfortunately, the lymphatic system doesn't have a pump, like the heart does, to push the fat and toxins it collects through it. So whenever you're detoxing, you must help the lymph system clear the toxins out. See Strategies for Eliminating Toxins (p. 136).

The Skin

While we usually think about our skin in terms of its appearance—whether we have zits or wrinkles, for instance—it's actually our body's largest organ. The skin coats our body, protecting us against infections; communicates vital information to our brain through the sense of touch; regulates body temperature; and functions like a second kidney. On top of helping with internal climate control, our sweat glands expel many toxins, especially under our arms (axilla region). Assuming our pores are open, the skin secretes over one pound of toxins each day. We know many of them as acne and blackheads.

But the pores on our skin can get clogged. Dead skin cells; residue from soaps, makeup and perfume, lotions and oils, powders and deodorants; and toxins and pollution are common culprits. When they become blocked, our skin can't breathe and excrete noxious substances. When pores stay blocked, we lose our ability to sweat, undermining the body's natural climate-control system, and trapping toxins and other impurities inside. That's why I'm not big on these lotions and potions with all these new additives— bronzers, shimmers, exfoliating agents, and so on—that people are now using. Some people's bodies are superb detoxifying machines and can handle them. After being damaged by all the toxicity, I know that mine is not. Even if my body were in better shape, I would not risk blocking my pores.

Strategies for Eliminating Toxins

The most effective way to eliminate harmful toxins is to have therapeutic detoxifying body treatments. While you're on the Martha's Vineyard Diet Detox, you should give yourself two detoxifying treatments every week, focusing on the body's primary organs of elimination: the colon, the liver, and the kidneys. There are two goals: One is to cleanse toxins out of your body at a rapid rate similar to which your cells are releasing them. The second is to help you learn what it takes to care for yourself, which few people understand because they're stressed out and overcommitted, and therefore neglect themselves. There are many, many detoxifying treatments. I've divided them into three categories: "must-have," "want-to-have" and "nice-to-have" if you have time and money. The "must-have" treatments are essential. Without them, toxins will back up in your body and you will feel terrible.

Providing much-needed support to your hard-working eliminatory organs, "want-to-have" treatments are great supplements to the "must-haves." Select a few of the "want-to-have" activities if you have time and money to do them, but many people will not, so I do not include them among the activities that are essential to this detox.

Must-have treatments:
- Water—six to eight cups (8 oz.) of distilled water daily
- Colonic
- Kidney flush
- Coffee enema

Want-to-have treatments:
- Chi machine
- Detoxifying bath
- Dry skin brush
- Rebounder (lymphatic drainage)
- Sauna

Nice treatments to get if you have time and money:
- Body wrap
- Cellulite treatment
- Ear coning
- Lymphatic drainage massage
- Gallbladder liver flush

Must-Have Treatments

Water

About 70 percent of the human body is composed of water. Without it we can't survive. While a person can live five weeks without food, they won't make it for five days without water. Why is it so important that we wet our whistle? H_2O aids our digestive processes; assists us in absorbing nutrients and transporting them throughout the body; aids our blood and other fluids in circulating; keeps our internal thermostat in check; and flushes out unwanted waste matter, fat, and toxins. We are constantly losing water when we urinate, move our bowels, and sweat, so we must drink water—not juice, not soda, not coffee—to replenish it. Just as water is vital to cleansing, nourishing, and lubricating the cells, it softens our stools and lubricates the colon, making it easier for our bowel movements to pass. Drink six to eight 8-ounce glasses of water (48 to 64 ounces total) daily while you're on the Martha's Vineyard Diet Detox. Again, you're drinking extra water while you're on the detox so it can help flush out cellular waste. If you do not drink the water, your results will be slower. Remember that the best water to drink during your detox is distilled.

Colon Cleanse

Not only does cleaning your colon help eliminate toxins that make you feel bad and cause you to gain weight, colon cleansing is an important technique to preserve your long-term, overall health. There are several ways to clean your colon, from drinking water to using herbal cleanse formula to giving yourself an enema to getting colonics. I recommend the following:

- *21-day detox:* three colonics (one per week), herbal-cleanse formula (daily)
- *7-day detox:* one colonic, herbal-cleanse formula (daily)
- *2-day detox:* herbal-cleanse formula (daily)

Colonics. Colon hydrotherapy is a way of cleansing the colon. I love colonics because they accomplish four things:

1. Soften the stool and flush out toxins
2. Soak the sludge (hard fecal matter), helping it to begin to slough off.
3. Lubricate the colon.
4. Retrain the colon to engage and improve peristalsis.

Colonics differ from enemas in that they have deeper cleaning power. The colon is approximately 5½ to 6 feet long and stretches to 2½ to 3 inches in diameter. There is enough water in an enema bag to stimulate peristalsis in the lower one-third of your colon. A colonic, on the other hand, can flush your entire colon out (whether this happens in any individual session has much to do with how impacted with feces it is).

Unlike enemas, which you can administer to yourself at home, colonics are administered by professionally trained *colon hydrotherapists* (colon therapists), experts in cleansing the colon and educating you on how that organ works. Find one by referral, and visit the website of the International Association for Colon Hydrotherapy (www.i-act.org) to make sure that they're certified.

When you get a colonic, you undress from the waist down and lie on a massage table, with your lower body covered by a sheet or towel. The colon therapist lubricates your anus with KY jelly or vitamin E oil, then slowly and gently slides the single leg of a hollow, Y-shaped speculum about an inch or two into your rectum. The speculum is about the size of a quarter. Since the rectum is a muscle designed to expand and contract, inserting the speculum doesn't hurt. However, anyone who has not done it before will experience different sensations than they may have experienced before. Although inserting the speculum can cause anxiety, it neither hurts nor feels particularly good. After a few moments, the rectum will relax and you may become unaware that the speculum is there.

The two branches at the wishbone-shaped end of the speculum are connected to two different hoses. The one attached to the narrow side of the Y directs a gentle stream of purified water into the body. Fecal material comes out through the other hose and empties into the sewage system.

To begin, the therapist opens the intake valve, allowing the colon to slowly fill. The patient feels his or her colon slowly filling with water, which softens the feces and loosens the sludge, making it easier for them to pass. To stimulate peristalsis, the therapist may alternate between admitting warm and cool water or may massage your abdomen. Eventually, the client feels the urge to have a bowel movement, at which point the therapist opens the outflow hose and the body's natural peristalsis propels the stool out of the body. The entire process is self-contained. When the client moves his or her bowels, there are no sounds, no smells, no spills, and no mess.

As the fecal matter exits through the outflow hose, it flows past a little window in the colonic machine on its way to the building's sewage system. This window in the machine acts as a window into your body, allowing you and the colon therapist to look at what's happening inside. The therapist can tell whether you're chewing your food well enough; if stool has become impacted into your colon's many nooks and crannies; whether your body is experiencing an overgrowth of *Candida* or yeast; if you have excess mucus, bacteria, toxins, or parasites.

Each patient's colon is rinsed and cleansed several times in each session. During the session, the therapist massages the stomach, helping to loosen impacted waste material and stimulate peristalsis. Over time, even a sluggish colon will "remember" how to contract, reducing the amount of time it takes to move waste out of the body. Depending on how impacted the client's colon is, the session can be more vigorous or extremely relaxing. Regardless, a colonic is an amazing educational session you truly never forget!

Afterwards, the colon hydrotherapist serves some *acidophilus* or another *probiotic* to help restore the good bacteria that live inside the colon. Immediately, you feel completely different—cleaner, lighter, and more energetic, true signs that your body was very toxic. It takes the average person three or more sessions to clean out the entire colon. By the third or fourth session the water might reach the cecum, the place where the large intestine starts.

Laxatives. The standard medical response when someone is constipated is to prescribe an over-the-counter or prescription laxative. There are several different types of laxatives, though people seem to prefer stool softeners and stimulants. I don't believe in using laxatives often. First of all, they're chemical stimulants, which means now you have more toxins in your bloodstream. On top of that, most laxatives irritate the colon, putting it into spasm and causing it to purge some—but not always all—of its contents. If you use them regularly, they can damage the colon without ever healing the root cause of why you're constipated in the first place. Many people become so accustomed to them that they unknowingly train their colon to be sluggish, rather than reconditioning it to engage in peristalsis. Consequently, when they don't take the laxative, they don't go to the bathroom. Finally, laxatives clean the inside of the colon out, but they don't slough off that sludgy fecal matter that lines your intestinal walls.

Rather than buying laxatives, I make colon-cleansing juices and teas at home. Here are some of my favorite—and most effective—concoctions. I've ranked them from Level 1, which provides a gentle cleanse, to Level 5 for people who are very constipated and have trouble moving their bowels.

Level 1: To 3 cups of water add 1 apple (chopped), 5 prunes, 5 figs, and stevia (to taste). Simmer with the lid on until the fruit is soft. Makes about 2 cups of juice. Drink. *Or* drink one ounce of whole-leaf aloe gel daily.

Level 2: Place one teaspoon of licorice root, one teaspoon of slippery elm, one teaspoon of crushed carob pod, and one teaspoon of flaxseed in a tea infuser and simmer in 2 cups of water for no longer than 2 minutes.

Level 3: To 2 cups of water add ¼ inch of a red hot pepper (not a red bell pepper), ⅛ inch of ginger root, and one clove of garlic. Simmer to taste. This tea can become very spicy hot, so drink with caution.

Level 4: Combine tea 2 with tea 3.

Level 5: Into one tea infuser place 1 teaspoon senna leaf, 1 teaspoon cascara sagrada leaf, and 1 teaspoon chamomile leaf. These ingredients can be found at an herb store. Simmer in 2 cups of water for no longer than 1 to 2 minutes, until water turns a light tea color. Drink one cup in the morning and one at night. *Note:* Do not use senna tea more than twice weekly. Senna is an irritant and can become addictive. It can begin to behave like a laxative, causing your colon to lose tone. But it's better to take senna than not to go at all!

Enemas. Many of our parents and grandparents regularly gave themselves enemas, a method of introducing water, herbs, coffee, or other active agents into your colon to soften fecal sludge and impacted stools, allowing them to pass out of the body. These days, enemas are less common. Even health care professionals do not give them anymore, which I think is a sin! Though many patients become constipated, health providers do not want to bother with a forty-five-minute procedure that requires dealing with your feces. They'd rather give you a laxative pill and a glass of water, though enemas are far more helpful.

Like your grandmother, you can give yourself an enema at home. You'll need the following supplies:

- One enema bag (disposable or hot-water-bottle style; purchase at a medical supply store or medically oriented pharmacy)
- 1 lemon *or* organic vinegar
- 1 gallon of distilled water
- 1 small bottle of vitamin E oil or 2 vitamin E capsules for lubrication
- 1 old towel or blanket
- 1 waterproof or plastic sheet

To do it you'll need to go to a medical supply store or medically oriented pharmacy and purchase an enema bag. There are two types of enema bags: the disposable, one-piece style or the old-fashioned hot-water red-bottle style. If you purchase a hot-water-bottle-style bag, instead of screwing a cap onto the top of the bag, you screw in the base of the long tube. At the other end of the tube you add on a thin applicator tip that you will gently slide into your rectum to introduce water into your colon. You'll also need one quart of distilled water. To this water add either the juice of one whole lemon or one tablespoon of organic vinegar. *Caution:* Do not go over this amount because both lemon juice and vinegar are acidic. The solution may become too strong for your sensitive inner colon.

Before you give yourself an enema, take a few moments to set up the room by lighting candles, burning incense, and playing soft music. You want to set a quiet mood. If you want to do it in the bathroom, place a plastic mat or blanket on the floor. You can also use your bed, if you place a plastic mat or waterproof sheet on top of it. If your bedroom is far from the bathroom, also line the floor with a protector in case you spill (or leak) any liquid. In order to avoid spills, make sure the applicator tip fits the tubing tightly, unless you have a one-piece disposable system, in which case this is not necessary. Make sure the clamp on the tubing is closed while you carry it. Also bring your vitamin E.

1. In your kitchen, pour the juice of one lemon or one tablespoon of the organic vinegar into your enema bag. Add one quart of lukewarm to room-temperature distilled water. (To ensure it is the proper temperature, test the solution on the inside of your wrist.) Screw on the top.

2. Carry the solution to your bathroom or bedroom. Hang the bag so that it is two feet above your head if you're lying down. The higher you hang the bag, the more pressure it exerts as it fills your colon, so hang it at a comfortable level.

3. Lubricate applicator tip with as much vitamin E oil as you need to insert it easily. You can also use olive oil or KY jelly.

4. Lie down on your right side and, to avoid spillage, insert the tip of the tube one to two inches into your rectum.

5. Release clamp, allowing water to gently enter your rectum. Count slowly to five (approximately half a cup of solution will enter the rectum), clamp bag. Repeat until all solution is used.

6. During and/or after taking in the solution, massage the lower left side of your abdomen. working on any hard lumps you may feel.

7. Retain solution for five minutes or until you feel a strong urge go to the toilet. If you don't feel the urge to purge, retain solu-

tion for up to fifteen minutes while massaging continuously. Then sit on the toilet and gently push the solution and waste matter out.

Liver Cleanse

If you have a poorly functioning liver, it affects your entire health. Fortunately, the liver is a very easy organ to cleanse. Here's what I recommend (see procedures for: coffee enema, juice flush and herbal remedies):

- *21-day detox:* three coffee enemas (one per week)
- *7-day detox:* one coffee enema
- *2-day detox:* one coffee enema

Juice Flush. We can flush the liver out merely by drinking green juices. Create any combination of these ingredients. Wheatgrass, however, should be consumed alone in one-ounce "shots."

- Wheatgrass
- Carrot
- Beets
- Beet leaves
- Dandelion greens
- Alfalfa sprouts
- Red radish or Daikon radish
- Burdock leaf or root
- Garlic
- Ginger

In addition, I recommend drinking herbal teas to help stimulate bile secretion and assist the liver to detoxify and repair its cells. Look for these ingredients:

- Barberry root bark
- Oregon grape root
- Beet leaf, burdock leaf and root
- Dandelion leaf and root

- Milk thistle
- Red clover

Coffee Enema. While a jolt of java gets us going in the morning, when introduced into the colon, coffee's caffeine can open up the bile ducts, stimulating the liver to release fat-emulsifying bile. It also stimulates the liver to produce glutathione, a very powerful antioxidant that causes the liver to cleanse our bloodstream. While we all have glutathione inside of us, as we get older and more toxic, the liver often secretes less of it. A coffee enema also helps the liver increase our glutathione levels, thereby stimulating a more efficient metabolism.

You administer a coffee enema very similarly to how you give yourself a regular enema. The major difference is that you cleanse yourself with organic coffee instead of organic vinegar or lemon juice. To prepare the solution, boil six to eight tablespoons of organic, ground coffee in approximately six cups of distilled water for no more than fifteen minutes. (*Note:* Decide how much coffee you're going to use based on how sensitive you are to caffeine. If you're very sensitive to caffeine, use four to six tablespoons; use eight tablespoons if you drink coffee often.) It is very important that you use distilled water; introducing tap-water toxins into your body just defeats the purpose of the enema. Spring water is better than tap water but not as pure as distilled. Allow the coffee to cool until it feels barely warm when you pour a few drops on the inside of your wrist. Carefully strain the solution to remove all the grounds. Unstrained coffee can clog up the tubing during the enema, causing a mocha mess. Pour the coffee solution into your enema bag, and then give yourself an enema, following the instructions described above.

Try to retain the coffee for five to fifteen minutes—but no more! If you retain coffee for too long, you may absorb too much caffeine and find yourself feeling wired and jittery. Don't worry whether you're a five-minute or fifteen-minute person; the point is to retain the coffee until you "gotta go, gotta go, gotta go, right now!" When you feel the urge, head to the bathroom. After you sit on the toilet, place your feet on a low bathroom stool, if you have one, and really push the feces and coffee out. This is the only time I ever teach people to push when they have a bowel movement. When you push during a coffee enema, your gallbladder opens, giving you the opportunity to cleanse your liver and bile ducts.

If you're like most people, after a coffee enema you'll feel exuberant and vibrant. You may feel like you love everyone! During your detox, you'll feel best if you perform a coffee enema once a week. Do no more than three during the 21-day protocol.

Kidney Cleanse

Flushing out the kidneys speeds our detoxification process by improving our blood flow and helping to regulate blood pressure. Anyone who has a tendency to retain water can benefit from a mild kidney flush to help keep the body fluids in balance and eliminate fluid retention.

- *21-day detox:* three kidney-cleanse drinks (one per week)
- *7-day detox:* one kidney-cleanse drink
- *2-day detox:* one kidney-cleanse drink

Black Cherry Kidney Flush. I used to drink this right before my period to help keep my stomach flat and to help keep me regular. Juice two bunches of fresh parsley; add ¼ cup black cherry juice, ¼ cup distilled water, then 5 drops of goldenrod tincture. If the taste is too strong, use less parsley. Drink only half a cup at a time followed by a warm cup of marshmallow root tea.

Want-to-Have Treatments

Chi Machine

My retreaters' favorite exercise, the Chi machine, helps detox your body as you lie flat on your back resting, reading, talking on the phone, or watching TV. You relax with your feet in the machine and it gently swings them back and forth, as though you were a fish in motion. By improving the movement of Chi (Qi), the

Chinese term for life-force energy, the exercise improves circulation, increases oxygen in the body, improves digestion, improves colon peristalsis, soothes tired muscles, eases joint pain, and helps to eliminate toxins. Because it takes stress off their body while assisting them with weight loss, I especially enjoy this exercise for people who are really heavy or obese, older, or very sedentary. It should be done daily and for up to an hour. Do this *or* the Rebounder (www.mvdietdetox.com).

Detoxifying Bath

Once a week prepare yourself a detox bath to help eliminate toxins and acid through your skin. Add the following to hot bath water: 2 cups of baking soda, which will help neutralize the acids contained in the toxins; 2 cups of Epsom salts, which gives the water a higher ion content than the body, drawing fluids and, therefore, toxins out of the body; a few drops of an essential oil, such as lavender for relaxation or peppermint for energy, so you benefit from the aroma therapeutic properties of the oils.

Dry Skin Brushing

By brushing your skin with a natural-bristled brush, you can help slough off your skin's outer layers so it can breathe and detoxify better. But don't do it the same way you slough your skin in the shower with a colorful plastic scrunchie. Brush your skin when it's dry instead, since this is the most effective way to remove the pore-clogging dead skin. The only implement you'll need is a vegetable-fiber bristled brush (not a loofah sponge, a sea sponge that is used wet, not dry, as a vegetable brush is) with a long handle to help you reach those hard-to-reach places.

For fifteen minutes brush your body in a circular motion, starting with your feet. The idea is to brush hard enough for your skin to become warm, rosy, and glowing, indicators that the top layers of skin are sloughing off. Next, take a hot shower followed by a cold shower. The hot shower relaxes and opens the skin's pores allowing toxins to escape; when you cool the water down, it closes the pores back up.

Lymph Drainage Massage

Unlike other types of massage whose goal may be to relieve muscular tension, a lymph massage is a technique to increase the flow of lymph, the fluid in the lymphatic system, helping toxins to be downloaded faster. To stimulate flow without harming surrounding tissues, the masseuse's touch should be very gentle. Benefits of a lymph drainage massage include reduced puffiness and swelling, a stronger immune system, healthier-looking skin, and greater relaxation.

Rebounder

Jumping lightly on a trampoline is one of the best exercises for detoxing. If you do it at least three times a week, it is an excellent way to stimulate and detox your lymphatic system. Jumping up and down improves the flow of fluid between the cells, which is why jumping on the Rebounder is often called cellular exercise. As you jump, the fluid moves out of the lymphatic system, decreasing excess fluid (edema) in the body, causing weight loss. Rebounding also helps circulate oxygen in the body, stimulates metabolism, improves coordination, enhances digestion, and strengthens the immune system. To start, begin bouncing once a day for ten minutes then increase slowly up to thirty minutes. If you want to bounce more than once a day, start at three to five minutes and slowly increase to fifteen minutes. Even if you do one or two minutes a day, rebounding can provide many internal health benefits. You can do this *and* the Chi machine daily in place of walking.

Sauna

One time for each week you're on the detox, try to sit in a sauna. Saunas help you lose weight by increasing your metabolism. They also rid the body of toxins, including heavy metals like lead, mercury, and nickel, and increase the flexibility of your muscles and joints. If you don't have access to a sauna through your health club or can't afford to go to a spa, check out your local YMCA/YWCA to see if you can buy a day pass.

Nice Treatments to Get If You Have Time and Money

Body Wrap

For each week you're on the detox, I suggest you give yourself a home detoxifying body wrap or get one at a spa. Body wraps are designed to take off inches rather than pounds. I like that you can concentrate on specific areas, such as heavy hips and thighs or a protruding abdomen. They also eliminate a myriad of toxins that have caused you to bloat and gain flab. To give yourself a wrap at home, soak Ace bandages (to cover your whole body, you'll need between twelve to fifteen and twenty to twenty-five bandages, depending on your size) in an herbal solution and wrap yourself up, apply a cellulite cream to your body and then apply the Ace bandages, or follow the procedure on the specific product that you purchase.

If you go to a spa they may use special mixes of herbs and mineral salts that slough off old skin, stimulate circulation, and reduce toxins; compression techniques; or products that actually penetrate the skin. If you feel bloated, overweight, or flabby, I suggest an Inch Loss Body Wrap. Your skin will feel tighter and firmer as the weeks pass. After a few treatments you will notice the bumpy appearance (cellulite) in your skin start to smooth out. For good results, have one body wrap per week.

Cellulite Treatments

As the skin ages, it begins to stretch and the space beneath it fills up and becomes clogged with excess toxin-filled fluid and fat cells, impeding the flow of blood and oxygen. When this happens, fat rises from the lower levels of the skin to the upper skin level, creating fat lobules (the dimple-like appearance beneath the skin). Eating foods that contain an overabundance of toxins, such as fried foods, alcohol, caffeine, salt, sugar, preservatives, and toxic chemicals, keeps the body from eliminating correctly, allowing these substances to build up in our fat cells.

Cellulite treatments are performed by first rubbing the area with a special cellulite cream that penetrates deeply into the skin, opening pores and allowing nutrients to penetrate and feed the skin. As this happens, the therapist applies specific movements, from percussion to vigorous palpation, circular movements, and pressure and stroking, to help dissolve lumps. To be effective these treatments must be performed by a skilled therapist. This therapeutic treatment should be done once per week or more for a time frame that varies with the treatment. Most people choose between cellulite treatments and body wraps.

The Gallbladder and Liver Flush

Cleansing the liver's bile ducts is a very powerful way to detox your liver; however, it is not for everyone (see below). Bile travels from the gallbladder through the bile ducts and into the liver. After you cleanse your kidneys, colon, and liver, it is important to cleanse this essential part of the system. This procedure will help to eliminate any liver crystals or stones in the gallbladder/liver system. Most people do this at the end of the detox, but you may choose to do it at any time after you've cleansed your other major eliminatory organs.

To prepare for this treatment, you must stop all herbal cleanse formula and kidney cleanse drinks the day before.

Note: If you have parasites or have chronic illness, DO NOT try this treatment. If you have parasites, this flush can actually stimulate their activity, causing them to move from one organ to the next, causing illness. You must check with your medical care provider before starting any treatments if you have a chronic or long-term illness.

This procedure requires the help of your colon therapist or a trip to the health-food store. It should only be performed toward the end of the 21-day detox, preferably on Day 19 and 20, with the colonic or Epsom salt flush taking place on Day 21. You will need the following ingredients:

- ½ gallon organic apple juice (*Note:* If you have diabetes, just use all water, no apple juice)
- 1 gallon distilled water
- 4 to 6 ounces cold-pressed olive oil

- 4 to 6 ounces of fresh-squeezed lemon juice (do not use lemon concentrate)
- 2 tablespoon Epsom salt (*Note:* If you have any chronic ill-nesses, consult with your colon therapist and health prac-titioner)
- 90 drops Superphos 30 Drops help to soften any gallstones that may be flushed out

There are at least five different ways of doing this particular liver flush, but the following is my preference:

Add ninety drops of Superphos 30 to a quart of organic apple juice. Some retreaters like to add ninety drops of Superphos 30 to a gallon of half distilled water and half organic apple juice in place of their other water for the day. This also helps to lessen the sweet-ness of the organic apple juice. Drink this for two days to soften any stones or hard crystals you may have in your gallbladder or liver. Right before bedtime on the second day, drink three ounces of fresh-squeezed lemon juice (about two to three lemons), mixed with three ounces of cold-pressed olive oil. Lie down on your right side for as long as possible.

In the morning you should have a colonic to remove stones. You may find gallstone-type objects in the stool ranging from light to dark green in color and varying in size (pea size to nickel size, sometimes larger; they may also be irregular in shape but mostly round, with a soft to moderately firm texture). If you are not hav-ing a colonic, then you may want to drink a solution containing one tablespoon of Epsom salt in one eight-ounce cup of water. Lie back down for two hours until you move your bowels or repeat the Epsom salt drink one more time.

7

SETTING UP FOR SUCCESS

Sherri had a beautiful designer kitchen in her suburban Chicago home. Not an appliance was out of place. She had a sparkling new, stainless steel Viking stove and refrigerator. Her cutlery was worthy of an executive chef. Her Italian marble counters were so spacious, clean, and clutter free that my son could have played air hockey on them. But Sherri didn't cook. I had come to stay with her for three weeks to help her lose weight and change her eating habits and lifestyle habits. As I opened her custom-made cabinet doors, toxin-filled food stared out at me, from bags of gourmet cookies and potato chips to cans of spaghetti and meatballs and pork and beans.

"This is not going to work," I told her.

"What's wrong?" she asked.

"You can't detox in this kitchen."

"Why not?"

"It's way too easy to fail in here, and I don't want you to waste your money," I told her. "We have to set you up so you can succeed."

With that I pulled out her trash can, climbed up on a stepladder, and started throwing food out: white-flour crackers, black beans, kippered herring, barbecue sauce, canned vegetables.

"But I paid good money for that food!" she cried.

"You're right," I told her. "You did pay good money for these toxins." I picked up an unopened bottle of her favorite salad dressing and read off the one or two natural ingredients on the label, followed by the long list of synthetic ones. Sherri's eyes got wide: "I didn't know all those chemicals were in there."

When she didn't try to stop me as I dropped it in the trash can, I knew that she knew she really needed my help.

"You have a choice," I said. "You can keep on putting poisons in your body, in which case there's no way you're going to lose weight, or you can decide, 'I'll just take the financial loss and chalk it up to experience. After I lose weight, I'll start over again with the right foods so I keep the pounds off.' "

She stood there with her mouth hanging open as I dropped canisters of powdered beverages, canned potato chips and onion rings, single-serving cans of fruit cocktail, an industrial-sized can of peaches drowning in high-fructose corn syrup, canned milk, and coffee creamer into the trash. To make a point I even threw in her can opener.

Then I opened her refrigerator and tore through the condiments. I tried to open the bottle of ketchup but couldn't—the lid was stuck shut. "When did you buy this?" I asked. Sherri couldn't answer. I asked the same of the mustard, relish, all the jams and jellies, horseradish, and bottled glazes and dips that lined her door and top shelf. She was shocked not to remember when she bought the food—and to realize how moldy some of it was. She said that some of the items had to have been sitting in her refrigerator for three years!

"You have to throw out old and toxic foods so you can replace them with good and healthy stuff," I told her as I poured her condiments down the drain. I knew that I was pushing our relationship, but with a fridge full of moldy food, what was she going to say? Before long, Sherri "got" what I was telling her and started to pitch in. When we finished, we pulled all her appliances out of the cabinets and set them out on the counter. Her kitchen wasn't quite as pretty, but it was definitely going to work.

When it comes to shedding pounds and maintaining healthy weight, "if you do not make a plan to succeed, you are going to succeed at failing." Since we live in a society that makes it unconscionably easy to make unhealthy food choices, the lure of our culture will pull you backwards unless you take bold and dramatic steps to resist it. To carry off the Martha's Vineyard Diet Detox, you will need to lay a foundation that's sturdy enough to support your transformation. My clients who prepare themselves in advance almost always achieve their goals. In fact, many exceed them. Those who don't set themselves up to win often find the change overwhelming. They run into obstacles and are not prepared to solve them, so they often find themselves getting sucked into old habits. Since you will need to make changes in your mind, body, and spirit, you need to prepare on all levels. Here, you'll find step-by-step instructions on how to begin.

Step 1: Plan Your Detox

Set Your Goals

You wouldn't embark on a trip without first deciding on a destination, purchasing your tickets, or looking at a map and filling your wallet with money. Nor should you begin the Martha's Vineyard Diet Detox without figuring out what you want to accomplish. Before you begin, set aside some quiet time to consider and answer questions like these in a journal:

- How much weight do I need to lose?
- Why do I want to lose weight? To fit my old clothes? Because I feel poorly? Is my health in jeopardy?
- Am I afraid that I'm going to get sick based on my current lifestyle or diseases that run in my family?
- Am I ready to make a permanent lifestyle change?
- Do I really believe that I should detox?
- What can detoxing do for me?
- How would detoxing change my lifestyle?
- Do I have the discipline to detox for 21 days or should I pick a shorter program?

Based on your thoughts and considerations, create some goals for yourself. Goals are the targets we shoot for, the end purposes we have in mind. Here are some goals other Martha's Vineyard Diet detoxers have set for themselves:

- To lose 21 pounds in 21 days
- To jump-start my 75-pound weight loss by losing 21 pounds in 21 days
- To improve my energy level
- To take every step in my power to reduce my blood pressure and sugar so I don't have to go on medication
- To detoxify from all the ways I abused my body while on vacation
- To detoxify so I can start my new healthy lifestyle with a clean body

Pick Your Program

Since life is dynamic and people are at different levels of commitment and ability, I am providing three options in hopes that you will find one that works with your lifestyle. Of course, I'm hoping that you dive right in and embark on the 21-day Detox so you experience the enjoyment of achieving maximum results. If you want to lose 21 pounds or to make major inroads in detoxifying your body and improving your health, you must detox for 21 days. To cleanse itself thoroughly, the body needs three weeks of rest from eating toxic food. During this time your body will remind you of how energetic you felt as a child. Your healthfulness will return. Your coworkers, friends, and family will compliment your looks. But if you, say, travel on business consistently or have a new baby or your life is generally unmanageable, you may decide that starting with the 21-day program may not be realistic. Kudos to you for being honest! There's no need to set yourself up to fail.

The fact that you don't feel capable of doing the 21-day Detox right now doesn't prohibit you from making significant progress toward changing your lifestyle to shed poisons and pounds. Consider following either the 7-day Tune-up or 2-day Weekend protocols. You *will not* lose 21 pounds if you follow either of these scenarios, but you *will* put important lifestyle changes in motion, begin cleansing and healing, and gain vital insider knowledge that will prepare you to detox longer later. Following the 7-day Diet Detox, you will be between five and ten pounds lighter, look visibly younger, feel more energetic, and experience increased overall wellness.

The Weekend Detox helps you improve your appearance and energy level quickly. Your eyes and skin will brighten; your thoughts will be clearer; you'll feel less stressed out, frustrated, and angry; and any allergies you experience will improve. If your body isn't tremendously toxic, you may lose between one and two pounds. If you turn the Weekend Detox into a lifestyle and clean your body out, you'll notice yourself losing more weight over time. Most importantly, the Weekend Detox allows you to become comfortable and competent with the process, allowing you to springboard to greater weight loss later. So do what your mind, body, and spirit can handle. It's important that you feel safe, comfortable, and ready for change. I suggest detoxing the following number of days annually:

- 21 days one time per year, totaling 21 days
- 7 days four times per year, totaling 28 days, or
- 2 days every weekend, totaling 104 days

When you detox for a shorter period of time, it takes a longer time to achieve results. That's because each time you detox, your body ramps up into deeper and deeper cleansing processes. Even then, you cannot get the cleansing power from 104 days of weekend detoxes that you get from one 21-day detox. However, over time the light maintenance the Weekend Detox offers is very helpful. And even if you do the 21-day detox, I suggest picking one day a week as a detox day when you follow the program. Many people already naturally detox for a day or two a week; they find they just aren't hungry.

Once you settle on a program, I want you to understand that *you don't have to be perfect!* The less you stray, the more weight

> *Note:* It is important to discontinue the Martha's Vineyard Diet Detox at the 21-day mark, at which point most people will require more protein and essential fatty acids.

you'll lose and the healthier you'll feel. But if you have a strong desire to chew and want to eat a salad in the middle of your detox, DO NOT DO IT! Drink free cleansing soups instead. The most important idea is to treat yourself significantly better than you've done in the past. If you do this, you'll do right by your body.

Talk to Your Doctor

Especially if you suffer from any illness, it is always prudent to tell your doctor before beginning any detox. I'll tell you up front that when you do this, your doctor will probably become alarmed. Remember: medical doctors are not educated in weight loss, nutrition, or detoxification. Your physician may warn you that the body naturally detoxifies itself and does not need any assistance. And while it *is* true that the body is designed to detoxify itself, it was not designed to live in this toxic environment. It cannot remove many of these noxious substances without an intervention. For that reason, you are giving it assistance.

I suggest that you explain these concepts to your doctor; however, I can't guarantee that you'll allay her concerns, which amount to fear of the unknown and belief that if they don't know it, it must not be true.

1. You will be removing junk food from your diet and learning healthy new eating habits.
2. While you detox, you will nourish yourself by drinking fresh vegetable juices and antioxidant drinks.
3. One of the side effects of detoxing is that you will lose weight.

Put Your Support System in Place

Unfortunately, we live in a culture that tells us we should "go it alone," but because the power of our habits and culture are so strong, I encourage people to embark on any lifestyle change in the company of others who can support and reinforce them. Try to get the entire family or your coworkers involved. Have fun. Start on a Thursday or Friday. Try to wean yourself off of coffee, cigarettes, and junk food, starting at least two days before the detox.

Clean Your Kitchen

Your body is never going to get clean if you keep shoveling toxins into it. One of the best ways you can support yourself is by cleaning out your kitchen. Now, I realize that not everyone can open up the pantry door and throw all the junk food out. Your husband and kids may not appreciate reaching for the corn chips or Cap'n Crunch only to discover they've gone the way of the plate scrapings from the night before. You can, however, discard the items that tempt *you*—the cookies 'n cream ice cream, the cheesecake topped with those cute red cherries.

If you eat the standard American diet, you may be wondering where to begin. Surprisingly, salad dressings and meat marinades are among the most unhealthy items in the average American's refrigerator. Read the ingredients listing and compare the short list of natural ingredients to the much longer list of synthetic chemicals and preservatives. It's shocking. To think that sometimes we put these synthetic chemicals on top of organic vegetables and meats that we mindfully select! Next, throw out your canned items, processed foods like frozen meals, chips, dips, crackers, non-whole-grain cereals, and all old food items including leftovers. You should throw out anything containing common processed chemicals such as high-fructose corn syrup, partially hydrogenated oils, hydrolyzed vegetable protein, and monosodium glutamate. We encourage you to research harmful chemicals in food. One resource I like is the Foods Standard Agency that serves the United Kingdom (www.food.gov.uk).

When you're done, you'll have plenty of space to store your supplements and other foods you'll use to do the Diet Detox. Finally, you'll need to clear some space on the front door of your refrigerator, where you can hang the daily schedule you'll follow during your detox and record how well you're doing.

Countdown to Your Detox

Now that you've set objectives, picked your program, talked to your doctor, put a support system in place, and cleaned out your kitchen, you'll need to pick the time when you will start (here, labeled "T") and start shopping so that you're ready to succeed. Here are the common steps people take to prepare for the 21-day program:

T minus 2 weeks
- Order or shop for supplies and supplements.
- Shop for a juicer.
- Make appointments for colonics, massages, and other treatments.

T minus 1 week
- Shop for a Crock-Pot, Tupperware storage containers, Thermos, water bottle, and the like.
- Set up your kitchen for success.

T minus 2 days
- Purchase your vegetables.

T minus 1-day
- Cut up and prepare your vegetables, placing them in storage bags and containers.

T
- Congratulations on embarking on the Detox!

T plus one day
- Congratulations—you have made it through Day 1.

T plus two days
- On this third day of detox you should be shopping for more fresh vegetables.
- Prepare vegetables in individual containers for the next three days.

Step 2: Shop for Success

After you've cleared your kitchen of toxic foods, the next step is to shop for healthy foods that will support the goals you've set for yourself. As a rule, the most healthy foods are those in their whole, most natural, form. The less it looks like the original ingredient it was derived from, the more processed it is. For the purposes of this detox, we'll focus on purchasing vegetables, seasonings, herbal teas, and high-density nutritional supplements.

Create a Shopping List

Any nutritionist or dietitian will tell you that nothing is more likely to scuttle a healthy-shopping trip than going to the supermarket hungry or without a list. It's hard enough when you smell the sausage and cheese frying on the sample station when you haven't had anything to eat, but to be starving and without a list is a sure recipe for overeating and overspending—your worst nightmare and a supermarket executive's dream! So let's begin by constructing a list of the kinds of items you'll need to purchase. Vary the quantities based on how often you plan to shop and who else will be consuming them.

Vegetables
- White: garlic
- Brown: ginger
- Purple: purple cabbage, beets
- Red: tomato
- Orange: carrots, sweet potatoes, yams
- Yellow: summer squash or yellow squash
- Green: broccoli, celery, cilantro, collard greens, cucumbers, kale, parsley, Swiss chard

Fruits
- Lemon, lime, and orange slices (place in pitchers of water to give you flavored water)

Spices
- Unsalted seasonings
- Cayenne pepper
- Curry powder
- Cumin
- Oregano
- Rosemary
- Thyme
- Dill

- Cinnamon
- Clove
- Bay leaf
- Cardamom
- Basil
- Caraway
- Coriander
- Fennel
- Mint
- Mustard
- Saffron
- Sage
- Turmeric
- Vanilla

Herbal teas

- Buy and sip on your favorite herbal teas throughout the detox to help keep hunger at bay. Feel free to purchase any brand or flavor that does not contain caffeine. It *is* okay to drink green tea, which does contain a small amount of caffeine, because green tea contains so many antioxidants. You can also drink teas that help relieve constipation, reduce stress, and so on. Plan to drink tea all day.

Go Grocery Shopping

Take a trip to the grocery store in your area that has the best produce section. While you're on the diet, you'll want to consume the freshest fruits and vegetables—organically grown, if you can afford it—and as many different types of produce as possible. You'll also want to make sure you can find all the ingredients you need for whatever soups you plan to make. But be forewarned: the nicest supermarkets are also the ones that use the most advanced techniques to encourage you to eat while you're shopping and spend more money than you need to on items like the gourmet chocolate candies you find near the cash register. You'll have to exercise resolve not to follow the aroma of freshly baked bread, nibble the new brand of frozen samosas offered as samples, or eat the beautiful fruit torts and tiramisu at the gourmet dessert counter. So eat before you go, take a detailed shopping list, and shop the produce section by color, selecting foods of every hue to maximize the nutrients and antioxidants you eat.

- Shop the perimeter of the store, where the fresh foods are sold and there are fewer processed foods.
- Avoid the prepared soups and canned vegetables, where ingredients like butter, whole milk, trans fats, salt, sugar and artificial flavors are often used to make foods look, smell, and taste better.
- Read the labels of any prepared or processed foods you buy, minimizing the number of ingredients whose names you can't pronounce, look like chemicals, or you don't recognize as a food.

Hit the Health-Food Store

If you do not order your supplements over the Internet (www.mvdietdetox.com), you'll need to head to the health-food store to buy the following:

- Juicer
- Stevia (Remember: a tiny bit of stevia goes a long way.)
- Food enzymes (ninety capsules or tablets)
- Green drink (Remember: look for a brand that contains a variety of different vegetables, not just wheatgrass or spirulina.)
- Antioxidant berry drink (Again, pick a brand that contains a wide variety of berries and has a high ORAC [oxygen radical absorbance capacity] value.)
- Herbal Cleanse Formula for the colon and liver
- Protein drink with soy, rice, or almond milk base (if you don't want to lose weight)

Shop at the Mass Merchandiser, Department Store, or Discount Store

This is the best place to buy a Crock-Pot, Tupperware storage containers, Thermos, water bottle, and other nonfood supplies.

Step 3: Set Up Your Kitchen for Success

There are the sneakers you wear when you want to look cute and the sneakers you wear when you go to the gym. They're not the same shoe. One is for pleasure, the other gets the job done. The same thing is true with your kitchen. As beautiful as your kitchen may be, I want you to turn it into a working kitchen while you're on the Diet Detox. By "working kitchen" I mean one that functions in your favor as you strive to lose weight and stay healthy. I want you to start by pulling out some forgotten wedding and housewarming gifts: your blender, juicer, and food processor. Place them out on the counter. You're going to use them every day.

Organize Your Refrigerator

Our goal here is to make doing the detox as fun, easy, and well organized as possible. On the outside of your refrigerator (or on the outside of a prominent cabinet), tape a copy of your daily Diet Detox program.

Next, wash your vegetables with lemon or lime juice or a vegetable cleaner you buy at the store. Once they are clean, lay them out on dish towels or paper towels, and use a salad spinner or pat them dry (wet veggies spoil quickly). Cut up your remaining vegetables, separating them into glass or hard plastic containers or resealable plastic bags. I recommend organizing your vegetables by color group, which makes them easy to identify and find, and helps the refrigerator look bright, colorful, and appealing. You can use these vegetables to make juice each day.

Create flavored water by slicing chunks of fruit and placing the chunks in glass pitchers full of distilled water so you can see how colorful and appealing the water looks. Drink as much of this water as often as you'd like through the day, though no less than sixty-four ounces.

TIP

As you cut the vegetables, store leftover fragments in a plastic bag to use in soup preparation.

Set Up Your Counters and Cabinets

Start by filling your teapot with water and placing it on the stove so that it is ready for you to drink tea all day. Tea has become an art form these days. You can buy name-brand herbal teas at the grocery store or specialty loose teas at a gourmet tea or coffee shop. It doesn't matter which flavor or type you prefer as long as it doesn't contain caffeine—the exception being green tea. I heat up a pot of water and add it to a Thermos or tea maker to keep water hot all day and have a cup of tea first thing in the morning. Then I drink tea all day long, switching flavors so I don't get bored. Although tea also contains vitamins and minerals, drinking it will also help you consume enough water.

Try attractively stacking a few decorative mugs on a counter or small tray. Keep teas of all flavors handy, as well as a basket of lemons and limes. You can replace the sugar in your sugar bowl with stevia powder or packets. If you like to flavor your tea with lemon or lime, place slices in a covered glass dish. You can even make fresh lemon or lime tea by squeezing the juice into your cup and adding hot water. You may also choose to make hot tea by the pot or a pitcher of sun or iced tea. One of my favorite teas I call Indian tea. It contains four cups of water, one stick of cinnamon, four to five cloves, one tablespoon of fennel, four whole cardamom pods, and one-fourth of a whole allspice clove. Simmer for an hour or to taste. Then add stevia and organic vanilla extract to taste. This tea not only gives you energy, it is great for your stomach.

> **FAQ: If plastic is toxic, shouldn't I avoid plastic bags and food-storage containers?**
>
> **A:** Ideally, yes. The healthiest containers for storing your foods are glass or stainless steel. In reality, most people have hard plastic containers like Tupperware, which are the next safest type. Many people also use plastic bags, which outgas more toxins than glass, stainless, or hard plastic. But there is such a thing as too much change, so I encourage people to focus on their nutrition first. If either now or later you want to change the way you store your food, you can tackle that as a separate step once you've finished the detox and lost weight, and your new lifestyle habits are established.

On your stove, you want to keep a pot full of vegetables cooking (or a Crock-Pot simmering). This is what I call your "free soup." You can eat it anytime during the day when you're feeling hungry. You can make your favorite soup minus the salt, sugar, eggs, butter, milk, and alcohol, pumping up the seasonings to add extra flavor. I have suggested some flavorful recipes on pages 205–208. You can also sip on vegetable broth.

Now that your cabinets have more room in them, you may also want to carve out some space especially for your products that your family knows not to bother. Some of my clients set aside a specific shelf or set of shelves for their supplements. For example, they may put different flavors of protein powders on one shelf and their supplements on another. Once you go off the detox and go on your weight maintenance plan, you may decide to add shelves to store your whole grains, dried beans and peas, nuts and seeds, cooking oils, and so on.

Step 4: Set Up Your World for Success

Forget the idea of your morning vitamin sitting in the kitchen cupboard. You're going to be nourishing yourself all day long, so you need to set yourself up differently to make that routine work. Wherever you're going to be, that's where you should store your supplements. Place a small glass, dish, or plastic bag containing your supplements in the following places:

- On your nightstand.
- By the bathroom sink: Packets of green drink, aloe vera supplement. When you wash in the morning, make a green drink. When you clean up before bedtime, take your aloe vera.
- In your purse, briefcase, or computer bag: packets of green drink, stevia, and herbal teas.
- In your car's cup holder: Green drink in a bottle or antioxidant mix with water.
- On your desk at work: A dish containing supplements.

I always suggest that people set alarms in their house and create computer reminders to prompt them to take their nutrients throughout the day. (Remember: you want to eat every two hours or less.) I have clients who are salespeople or soccer moms and do a lot of driving. They won't leave home without their cooler in their car so the cleansing soups, green drinks, and fresh juice they made at home stay cold all day.

Eventually, as the visual cues take hold and you become accustomed to the program, these guidelines become automatic.

Step 5: Plan Your Day

I like to encourage my clients to plan for two types of days: days they will spend at work and those they'll spend at home. They require two different types of preparation and organization.

Work Days

Because you will not have ready access to your supplies at home, days when you're working and/or traveling will require additional preparation. Fortunately, the program is very flexible, there are juice bars all over the country (except on Martha's Vineyard!), and many chefs will even cook to your specifications. Even though we live in a toxic environment, a lot more resources are available than before for those of us who want to eat healthily.

But a lot of people tell me, "I can't juice at work! It requires too much equipment. It's too messy!" Fortunately, you don't need to. You can substitute your green drink and antioxidant berry drink for juice. Just pour some directly into a small bottle of water or take it with you in a baggie, pour it into a water bottle, and shake it up at work. Some of my clients even buy portable blenders to mix their supplement drinks. If you purchase a Thermos, you can take your soup or broth with you. Many of the most successful people even keep a set of supplies at the office.

Home Days

Follow the daily schedule provided on page 174.

Testimonial

JUDI THOMPSON

Age: 44
Family status: married mother of teenaged twins
Occupation: flight attendant
Location: Houston, Texas

I have been a flight attendant for twenty-three years, but once I turned forty, I started having trouble losing the five pounds that I used to lose with the wink of an eye. I had been a size 6–8 and liked to stay anywhere between 121 and 130 pounds, but my weight had climbed above and beyond 140 and there was no stopping it. I had become a size 10–12. I didn't know what was going on, so I tried those quick-take-off diets. They didn't work. I'd lose a little, then gain a lot back. I despise exercising, so I had an additional strike against me. In my profession, I remember the days of weigh-ins and being put on a probation period when one didn't meet the height to weight restrictions, so I always tried to stay proportionate and look neat and polished in my uniform. After all, I wasn't only representing myself, but the image of a professional airline.

James Hester introduced me to the diet. Over the years I had watched him change from being a very handsome man to become very overweight and sluggish looking. He really let himself go (I can say these things because he is my brother). Then, he experienced this miraculous weight loss. Eight weeks after I'd seen him last, my family visited him in New York for the holidays. When he walked up to me on the busy street, I paused. He looked different, younger and more vibrant than I had ever seen him. He was so amazingly gorgeous. His body looked toned and fit. His skin glowed. He looked like he had undergone serious cosmetic surgery. I couldn't keep my eyes off of him! Next, I noticed how much energy he had. I couldn't wait to hear how he accomplished this transformation so quickly. He then told me his little secret and offered to assist me in losing my weight, but said it wouldn't be easy. So he asked me to think about it and when I was ready to make the commitment, he'd come down to Texas and get me started. We have a motto in our family "What we start, we must finish," so I didn't call him for quite a few months. Then I made up my mind that I was going to go through with it and there was no looking back. James arrived on a Friday and we got started right away. He helped me for the first ten days and was a tough but very loving coach.

Once I started the detox, I was shocked that I was rarely ever hungry. I love food; I love to chew. I go to these wonderful places around the world where there's amazing food and amazing restaurants—I should weigh about 200 pounds considering how much I enjoy eating. But while I was on the detox, I kept myself to the regimented schedule and drank tons of water to prevent unwanted hunger pangs. Even when I made my family their regular daily meals, I wasn't tempted to join them. I'd prepare my green drink and be very satisfied until the next meal came two hours later. Have you ever fasted for a number of weeks and given up the things that you really love to eat, like bread, sweets, flour, good wine, alcohol? It's really the same mind-set. Our mind will work for us favorably if we allow it to.

I have an extremely active family life and my job requires me to travel; therefore, if this detox was going to work in my favor, it had to be portable. Every three days I would go shopping at Whole Foods or Central Market HEB, get enough organic veggies for three days, then clean and slice them and put them into Ziploc bags. That way, I would have them in my crisper all ready to go. It took approximately twenty to thirty minutes each morning to set myself up for the day. If I was going out that day, I'd make two green drinks and Regenicare (a lemon-tasting supplement), put them in water bottles, and head out for the day. Whether I was out running around town or driving my sons to basketball practice every day, the bottles were in a cooler on ice ready to shake up and drink. I would also always have at least a gallon of distilled water with me at all times. My goal was to drink a gallon of water a day. Most days, I achieved my goal. When evening came, I'd take the bags of cut-up veggies out of the fridge, boil them down and puree them, and add a dash of spice to enhance the flavor a bit. It was really that easy.

For the last eleven days, the detox came on the road with me. I fly all around Europe in and out of different time zones. This time I had one trip scheduled for London and one the following week to Paris, but I made a commitment to stay on schedule. So everywhere I traveled, I'd go online and Google live juice bars, then Mapquest the location from my hotel. I discovered that there is a juice bar right at the Gatwick airport. So how easy is that? When I was in Paris, by no coincidence, the nearest juice bar was just five minutes away from where I stay. I would get my juice in the morning or a wheatgrass shot during the day and be good to go! In addition to drinking fresh juice, I would take all my products in Ziploc travel-size packets on the road with me. I purchased a battery-operated blender and carried it in my suitcase. Toward the end of the detox, I prepared the soup in advance and froze enough to last for five days. James and Dr. Roni told me that it's better for you when it's fresh, but given that I was on the road it had to work.

A person who is very, very active in his or her life can take the diet on the road and have successful results. It is all about making the commitment to succeed—seeing the 21 days as a goal and not stopping until you reach it. I am living and breathing proof that it works if one is willing to do the work.

After 21 days of detoxing, I did lose 16 pounds and two inches. I had an incredible amount of energy. Prior to detoxing I suffered from restless leg syndrome and took Aleve every day for relief. Not one time did I have to reach for the Aleve. My legs never felt better. My legs were thinner and more toned, my waist and bustline decreased, my crow's feet and frown marks on my forehead started to disappear, my hair and skin looked shiny and healthy. I got back to a size 8, and had never felt healthier in my life. Dr. Roni suspected that I did not lose 21 pounds because I was perimenopausal, so I went to the doctors and had blood taken and discovered that I may be. She also suspects that some infertility medications I took many years ago might be interfering with weight loss. Recently, I underwent a major operation to remove a six-pound tumor from my uterine wall. That, too, could've blocked my success path to my total weight loss results. Bottom line: my body desperately needed to detox. I learned that if you're not losing weight the way the diet suggests, a health problem may be getting in the way.

So was the Martha's Vineyard Diet Detox easy? No, it was not. Was it something I enjoyed doing for 21 days? To be honest, I didn't love it. But I didn't love being 25 pounds overweight either, and the older I get, the harder it is to lose weight easily. The detox can become a lifestyle for some people; however, I'm not one of those people. But I am definitely committed to detoxing two to three times a year. It was such a rewarding challenge to get healthy from the inside out. And I did like the results very much. I got more rewards than just weight loss; I discovered the benefits of feeling healthy. It's really awakened my metabolism. I am not sluggish any longer; I always have energy and I always feel good.

At times, I do return back to my old eating habits, but I'm not as indulgent as in the past. I want to keep looking and feeling as good as I do right now for a long time to come. Taking the toxins out of my body really helped me. I would definitely recommend this detox/diet to anyone who seriously wants to address their toxic eating habits and desires an opportunity to get healthy and stay that way.

8

DOING THE DETOX

Now that you understand the principles behind the detox, you're ready to get started. Because the program is detailed, I'm providing you with daily and weekly plans to follow. They describe activities that are essential as well as those that are optional. For instance, you'll feel really lousy and it will slow your weight loss if you don't get a colonic, or at least do a water enema. While a body wrap helps you detox and you'll feel better if you do it, it is less powerful, so it is optional. Use the information in this chapter as a guideline, not a prescription. However, it is essential that you follow the daily schedule, not just because it helps you detox most efficiently, but because it keeps you from feeling hungry, which helps ensure you'll stay on the plan and meet your weight-loss goals.

I also want you to remember that this is not an all-or-nothing program. I encourage you to choose the detox that works best for your goals and lifestyle. Each will give you results. Also, at any time you want, you can eat free soup. Remember, free soup is designed to give you minerals and fluids and a strong taste that will take the edge off of any hunger you may feel. It is best not to chew anything, since chewing reactivates your digestive process, which we are intentionally putting on hold to convert the digestive energy to healing. Whatever your personal reason for detoxing, why not use what you've learned to begin to implement lifestyle changes now? You're setting yourself up to live a healthier, more energetic life.

> The daily schedule is the same whether you do the 21-day Diet Detox, the 7-day Tune-Up, or the 2-day Weekend Cleanse.

Daily Supplement Schedule

8:30 A.M.
- high-density antioxidant berry drink
- herbal cleansing formula
- 1 cup hot herbal tea (lemon and stevia optional)
- 8-ounce bottle of water

10:30 A.M.
- 8-ounce bottle of water with high-density green drink mixed into it
- 8-ounce glass of hot or iced herbal tea (lemon and stevia optional)

12:30 P.M.
- 1 cup fresh vegetable juice (choose mostly green vegetables, but add a little carrot or beets for sweetness if you like). If you're not juicing, then consume another high-density green drink.
- 1 enzyme capsule (consume only if you juice; most green drinks already contain enzymes)
- herbal cleansing formula, according to the instructions on the label
- 8-ounce bottle of water

2:30 P.M.
- 8-ounce bottle of water
- high-density green drink
- 8-ounce glass of hot or iced herbal tea (lemon and stevia optional)

4:30 P.M.
- high-density antioxidant or berry drink

6:00 P.M.
- 1 cup homemade cleansing soup
- 1 cup broth from cleansing soup mix
- 1 cup of your favorite herbal tea
- 1 enzyme capsule
- herbal cleansing formula, according to the instructions on the label
- 8-ounce bottle of water

7:30 P.M.
- 8-ounce cup of hot or iced herbal tea (lemon and stevia optional) or 8-ounce bottle of water

Bedtime
- aloe vera

* Please check with www.mvdietdetox.com for changes and supplements.

Avoiding the Danger Zone

If you wait longer than two hours between eating, you may find yourself feeling a little hungry. This is when you're most at risk for not only breaking your detox, but doing so in a way that may make you gain a lot of weight and jeopardize your health.

When you detox, cells all over your body are new and wide open. You've turned back the clock so that your gastrointestinal (GI) system is almost as pure as a newborn baby's. You must transition it slowly into a diet of mixed foods, just as you prepare the digestive system of a baby to break down different types of foods, starting with rice cereal and slowly building from there.

Since your cells are so clean and new, if you suddenly put toxic foods into your system, you will feel much worse than before you started. You can even make yourself sick. If you eat foods that are very toxic, you can send your body into anaphylactic reaction, a severe allergic reaction that occurs when the body is exposed to a specific allergen or toxic substance. Examples of anaphylactic reactions include people who have trouble breathing after tasting or smelling nuts or seafood. Worst case, their airway closes and they can't breathe and can die. This is a particular risk when you've cleaned out your system, yet go off the detox incorrectly. Whatever you do, if you cheat, don't drink alcohol, smoke cigarettes, take illegal drugs, eat a fast-food meal, or pig out on junk food. Eat vegetable cleansing soups, fruit, or salad instead. If you decide to discontinue your detox, you must transition back to a mixed diet by following the process described in Chapter 9.

21-Day Cleansing Treatment Schedule

In addition to following the hourly nutritional schedule, it's essential to engage in daily activities to remove the toxins you flush from your cells out of your body altogether. These activities, which are described in detail in Chapter 6, are depicted in the chart below. Since people's budgetary and time constraints vary, I have designated these activities as must-have (M), want-to-have (W), and nice to do if you have time and money (N). I strongly encourage you to do the must-have activities. Skipping them may cause you to feel poorly and even to become sick. The more cleansing treatments you are able to do, the faster you will flush the toxins out. Consequently, the better you'll feel. Though you are still likely to experience a healing crisis, it will be milder and shorter in duration. If your healing crisis feels uncomfortable, reread "Riding Out the Healing Crisis" on page 89.

Day 1

M—Colonic: schedule in advance with colon therapist

M—Walk one mile at leisurely pace or use the Rebounder for 20 minutes

W—Brush dry skin before showers

N—Chi machine

Day 2

M—Walk one mile at a leisurely pace or use Rebounder for twenty minutes

W—Brush dry skin before showers

W—Lymphatic drainage massage

N—Chi machine

Day 3

M—Coffee enema: see procedure on pages 145–146

M—Walk one mile at leisurely pace or use Rebounder for twenty minutes

W—Brush dry skin before showers

N—Chi machine

Day 4

M—Walk one mile at leisurely pace or use Rebounder for twenty minutes

W—Brush dry skin before showers

N—Body wrap

N—Chi machine

Day 5

M—Walk one mile at a leisurely pace or use Rebounder for twenty minutes

W—Brush dry skin before showers

N—Cellulite treatment

N—Chi machine

Day 6

M—Kidney cleanse drink

M—Walk one mile at leisurely pace or use Rebounder for twenty minutes

W—Brush dry skin before showers

W—Detoxifying bath

N—Chi machine

Day 7

M—Walk one mile at a leisurely pace or use Rebounder for twenty minutes

W—Brush dry skin before showers

W—Sauna treatment

N—Chi machine

Day 8

M—Colonic

M—Walk one mile at leisurely pace or use Rebounder for twenty minutes

W—Brush dry skin before showers

N—Chi machine

Day 9

M—Walk one mile at leisurely pace or use Rebounder for twenty minutes

W—Brush dry skin before showers

W—Lymphatic drainage massage

N—Chi machine

Day 10

M—Walk one mile at a leisurely pace or use Rebounder for twenty minutes

W—Brush dry skin before showers

N—Body wrap

N—Chi machine

Day 11

M—Coffee enema

M—Walk one mile at a leisurely pace or use Rebounder for twenty minutes

W—Brush dry skin before showers

N—Chi machine

Day 12

M—Walk one mile at leisurely pace or use Rebounder for twenty minutes

W—Brush dry skin before showers

N—Cellulite treatment

N—Chi machine

Day 13

M—Walk one mile at a leisurely pace or use Rebounder for twenty minutes

W—Brush dry skin before showers

W—Detoxifying bath

W—Sauna treatment

N—Chi machine

Day 14

M—Walk one mile at a leisurely pace or use Rebounder for twenty minutes

M—Kidney cleanse

W—Brush dry skin before showers

N—Chi machine

Day 15

M—Colonic

M—Walk one mile at a leisurely pace or use Rebounder for twenty minutes

W—Brush dry skin before showers

N—Chi machine

Day 16

M—Kidney cleanse drink

M—Walk one mile at a leisurely pace or use Rebounder for twenty minutes

W—Brush dry skin before showers

W—Lymphatic massage

W—Sauna treatment

N—Chi machine

Day 17

M—Coffee enema

M—Walk one mile at a leisurely pace or use Rebounder for twenty minutes

W—Brush dry skin before showers

N—Chi machine

Day 18

M—Kidney cleanse drink

M—Walk one mile at a leisurely pace or use Rebounder for twenty minutes

W—Brush dry skin before showers

N—Body wrap

N—Chi machine

Day 19

N—Start gallbladder and liver flush

M—Walk one mile at a leisurely pace or use Rebounder for twenty minutes

W—Brush dry skin before showers

N—Cellulite treatment

N—Chi machine

Day 20

N—Continue gallbladder and liver flush

M—Walk one mile at a leisurely pace or use Rebounder for twenty minutes

W—Brush dry skin before showers

W—Detoxifying bath

N—Chi machine

Day 21

N—Colonic to end gallbladder and kidney flush

M—Walk one mile at a leisurely pace or use Rebounder for twenty minutes

W—Brush dry skin before showers

N—Chi machine

Trouble-Shooting Tips

Sometimes even the most conscientious detoxers have trouble losing weight. Some people lose several inches while detoxing, but significantly fewer pounds than they would like. Others experience times when they are not losing weight because the weight of the fat they are shedding is offset by increasing muscle mass, which weighs more than fat. While there are many reasons why people experience slower-than-normal weight loss (see list in Chapter 1), they often experience similar symptoms, including:

- Chronic bloating and gas after eating
- Sugar and carbohydrate cravings
- Constipation or diarrhea
- Chronic fatigue or tiredness upon waking
- Extreme feelings of hot or cold

- Feeling bad after taking medications or experiencing side effects
- Depression and anxiety
- Food cravings after quitting smoking

If you are experiencing any of these symptoms, these home remedies may reboot your weight loss. However, you may need to consult with your health care provider to determine if you are having a thyroid problem or hormone imbalance that may require more serious intervention.

- Intestinal discomfort: Extra enzymes or an aloe vera supplement.
- *Candida:* Yeast imbalances can cause sugar or carbohydrate cravings. To identify whether you have one, take a *Candida* test at an alternative practitioner's office. If your test returns positive, you'll need to add protein shakes to your detox; drinking too many juices with too many complex carbohydrates will just feed the yeast or slow your weight loss.
- Excessive cravings: Sugar-controlling herbs such as Glucofast, which is especially good if you are insulin resistant. You will have a hard time finding Glucofast at the health-food store; instead, go to www.mvdietdetox.com.
- Constipation: See a colon therapist or take the detox and cleansing tea daily in addition to the liver and colon herb formula.
- Fatigue: Try kelp or dulse (seaweed type of vegetable) that you add to cleansing soups, which give the body extra minerals, sodium, and iodine. If you feel most fatigued after exercise, you may need additional minerals, as described in Chapter 5.
- Extreme body-temperature changes: If you experience hot flashes, feel cold all the time, or have cold extremities, ask your medical provider to perform a hormone panel to evaluate your hormone levels. If you feel your menstrual cycle

is interfering with weight loss, try applying progesterone cream. It can also be useful for treating hot flashes. If you are cold all the time, ask your doctor if you need a thyroid panel.

- Depression: If you are taking antidepressant medication, see your health care provider. If not, try adding essential fatty acids and protein drinks containing amino acids to the detox. This will help relieve the depression, but will slow the weight loss associated with this detox.
- Prescription drugs sometimes prevent you from losing weight. Some actually cause you to gain weight. If you suspect this is happening to you, consult with your medical care provider to discuss your alternatives.
- Sluggish metabolism: If you feel that your metabolism has slowed down due to a hormonal imbalance or if you have insulin resistance, try Glucofast (see above).
- Smoking: Is one of the reasons you smoke to keep your weight down? If so, you need to increase your exercise. Take on a sport or join the gym to keep your mind off smoking and eating.
- Parasites: If you have had parasites in the past or suspect you have them now; experience chronic bloating, gas, or indigestion; or travel frequently, particularly internationally, I suggest that you drink the following parasite-preventing tea daily during your detox (you must go through a parasite cleanse to get rid of active parasites). It is called Indian Tea.

Ingredients:
4–5 whole cardamom pods
½ stick cinnamon
2 tablespoons fennel seeds
10 whole cloves
5 drops black walnut tincture (found at health-food store)
1–2 packets of stevia
Vanilla and/or almond extract, to taste (optional)

Break the shells of the cardamom pods to release the spice and strengthen the tea's potency. Boil spices in a quart of water, until the tea tastes strong. After boiling, you may add a teabag of your favorite tea, such as chamomile, to enhance the flavor. Add a packet or two of stevia. Simmer. Remove from heat and add 5 drops of black walnut tincture. Add vanilla extract or almond extract to taste (you can also modify the herbs to strengthen the taste). Drink.

Testimonial
HILARY BEARD

Age: 44
Occupation: writer and editor
Location: Philadelphia

Two days before I received the first phone call about being the writer on this book project, I asked God to help me with my fibroids. I've had fibroids for twenty years. Over the previous six months my period had gotten heavier, and earlier in the year I had experienced a very heavy period that came after only two weeks. EEEK! My gynecologist suggested birth control pills or surgery, neither of which I wanted to pursue. So when James called inquiring whether I might be interested in working on this project, I knew God was sending my answer!

I was excited about detoxing my body. I've detoxed twice—I did a water fast for three days about ten years ago. It was miserable. When I'm hungry I can't sleep, so I get overly tired and feel like a kid on the verge of a temper tantrum. I've also done the Master Cleanse (the Lemonade Diet) for four days. I liked it because I didn't feel hungry. The only problem was, I didn't have a plan. Halfway through the fifth day, I ran out of maple syrup and crashed. Hard. So hard that I bought a Mrs. Smith's blueberry pie and ate it, defeating the point of the detox. I experienced by far the worst breakout of my life—I looked like a pimply teenager. I'm lucky I didn't get sick. So I welcomed the idea of being detoxed by a pro. I aspired to do the 21-day detox—but I didn't want to feel hungry and I didn't want to lose weight. I decided to work up to it in stages—doing the weekend detox first, then the 7-day. I'd conquer the 21-day program last.

I did a three-day detox at the Inn. I figured that since I had once survived on water for three days, it shouldn't be too bad. Still, I didn't want to be hungry. Dr. Roni promised I wouldn't be. I wasn't sure I believed her, but I decided to give the Detox a try. She was wrong; it took a couple of days for her and Linda Hicks, another naturopath on staff, to figure out how much nourishment I needed. Apparently I have a fast metabolism—sometimes I'd find myself feeling slight hunger pangs as soon as fifteen minutes after being fed. Dr. Roni first eliminated digestive enzymes, which I clearly didn't need. That helped a lot but didn't solve the problem. Linda started feeding me protein shakes, which meant that I was no longer on the strict detox, though my body was clearly cleansing. Protein shakes helped a lot, but I still found myself sneaking into the kitchen in the middle of the night to make myself a shake. She started adding essential fatty acids to my shakes.

During the detox I didn't feel tired and I was never uncomfortably hungry even though we were adjusting my portions. I'm healthy and take good care of myself, so I didn't experience any memorable healing crisis or anything unusual. I just peed an awful lot. I reluctantly accepted Dr. Roni's suggestion that I not wear any deodorant so my body could cleanse through my underarms. I felt sensitive about my hygiene, but her explanation made sense so I figured I'd try it and wash up a lot.

At the end of the three days, I could tell that my system was cleaner than usual. I had lost a few pounds, which I wasn't happy about. I had urinated so much I figured it was probably water weight. But it wasn't like I had slowed my pace, as a normal retreater might, so what did I expect? After completing three days I returned home, thinking everything was normal. I was wrong. Over twenty people told me how great I looked! People I knew and people I didn't know commented on the appearance of my skin. Something had changed that was obvious to everyone. What a pleasant surprise!

I carried the momentum from the detox into the next month's lifestyle habits at home. I figured that I'd prepare fresh vegetable juice on as many days as I could as a nutritional supplement to my regular meals. I was so enthused that I juiced on twenty-seven out of thirty days. Over that month, even *I* had to admit that my skin looked amazing! After about two and a half weeks of daily juicing, I started waking up at 4:30 A.M., unable to get back to sleep. I wracked my brain trying to figure out the reason for my sudden insomnia. Then it dawned on me that I wasn't tired. Dr. Roni had told me the detox would give me more energy. I had assumed she'd meant I'd feel perky and peppy. That hadn't happened. For me, more energy meant more waking hours. By the end of that month, I had picked up two additional hours of awake time in the morning and three or more hours of alert time in the evening because I stopped snoozing in front of the TV and was wide awake until midnight. All this from improving my nutrition? I couldn't believe it! I remembered that when I was in my twenties, I had had enough energy to work all day, then eat and run my errands, then go to the gym at 10:00 at night. That's how I felt after my detox. I hadn't had this much energy for twenty years. I couldn't believe how, as healthy as I thought I was, my quality of life had declined in such small increments that I hadn't noticed it!

Next, I tried the 7-day Detox, also at the Inn, where Roni and I were working on this book. I was confident that I could complete the 7 days, but the specter of the 21-day lurked in the back of my mind. I really wanted to do it, but couldn't imagine myself succeeding. I stopped talking about it with friends and family because I didn't want to speak myself into failing. First things first, I thought. Just do the 7 days.

Two days into my 7-day Detox, Linda cracked the code on how to keep me from feeling hungry. Over the week she supplemented my protein shakes with ingredients ranging from a dollop of plain yogurt to sesame tahini to coconut milk to avocado. She also added ghee to my dinner cleansing soups. Ghee is clarified butter from which the water and milk fat have been removed. It is frequently used in Indian and South Asian cooking. I felt much better. The nourishment I was receiving finally "stuck to my ribs." At this point I was way off the program, but I didn't care. I was doing something much better for myself than I had ever done in my life. What did it matter if I wasn't following the rules to the letter?

On Days 1 and 2, I felt great and I began to see the pores in my face cleaning themselves out again. I decided to follow Roni's suggestion and not wear any deodorant. On Day 3 I coughed up a lot of mucus—so much that it disrupted my sleep. I kept feeling like I was going to choke on all the mucus that was draining into my throat. I also noticed my ears itching. Where did all that wax come from? I developed matching zits on both sides of my neck, followed by matching zits on each side of my forehead. All over my body my skin started to shine and glow. The skin on my lower legs was no longer dry. My heels, which are usually a little bit on the dry side, were hydrated and as soft as my hands. Could the dry skin I had suffered from since childhood merely be a nutritional imbalance? Apparently so.

On Days 4 and 5, I found myself feeling sad—not sad enough to cry; however, something I couldn't put my finger on was definitely bubbling up. On the night of Day 5, I started crying—I'm still not sure what about. I cried for maybe an hour, but then it was over and I felt fine. Day 6 went wonderfully. I knew I'd be driving home the next day and wanted to continue the detox for another couple of days—I hadn't thought about how many. Since I'd be traveling for eight hours, Linda helped me figure out how to get through the day. We made a protein shake the night before, poured it into a water bottle, and put it in the freezer. I would sip on it as it defrosted during the drive. We put a bunch of celery, carrots, and radishes in a baggie. Roni made some kind of cucumber/soy/ginger dressing that I poured over them. I nibbled on them on the ride home. I stopped at McDonald's along the way and picked up an Asian salad—hold the chicken. More cheating, but given my fast metabolism I needed it.

As soon as I got home, I headed straight for the grocery store to stock up on organic vegetables so I could detox for a few more days. By this point I knew that if I didn't have my supplies, I was in danger of crashing and coming off the detox the wrong way. After working with Dr. Roni, I understood the importance of breaking the detox correctly. That night I decided to use my Crock-Pot for more than decoration. For the first time in five years I threw a bunch of vegetables into it—kale, collards, carrots, yellow squash, zucchini, red pepper, green pepper. Even though kale and collards didn't fit the menu, I figured I'd make an Italian-flavored cleansing soup. I seasoned it with oregano, rosemary, basil, and pepper and cooked it overnight. That was easy enough. It tasted great. I had survived Days 8 and 9.

But on the evening of Day 9, I ran into a crisis. It was 9:00 P.M., I was hungry, out of cleansing soups, and there were hardly any vegetables left in my fridge. I had purchased more veggies than I'd ever eaten before. Where had an entire refrigerator full of vegetables gone in two days, I wondered? The answer—I had consumed them—gave me a reality check on how many veggies you run through when you're making pureed cleansing soups. A Crock-Pot crammed with vegetables might reduce down to a quart of pureed cleansing soups—plus, I was juicing, which consumes a lot of vegetables. I realized I'd have to go shopping daily—or at least every other day. That night I "cheated" and ate a salad for dinner. I went shopping first thing on Day 10. I bought vegetables along with some grains and fruit so I could begin to go off my detox beginning the next day. But when the next day came, I didn't want to go off the detox. I figured I'd try to make it to the 14-day mark. On another day I went too long between "feedings." I could feel myself crashing. I cheated again by eating a vegetarian platter from a Middle Eastern restaurant. When I got to 14 days, I didn't want to go off. Even though I wasn't doing the hardcore detox because I didn't want to lose weight, I had almost made it to 21 days. I had boatloads of energy; I might as well keep going! My skin looked amazing; my fingernails had gotten very hard—so strong that they didn't break or chip when I traveled with luggage (traveling is often hard on my nails). And they were growing so fast I had to trim them twice a week.

At that point I figured I'd better get a colonic. I had known that detoxers were supposed to get one colonic a week. I had gotten one colonic and one coffee enema during that first week with Dr. Roni. When I tried to make an appointment with the woman who had been giving me colonics for over ten years, I couldn't get in until the equivalent of Day 25. That meant I had to consider giving myself an enema. EEW! I hate to sound like a snob, but in this area I am: I'd rather pay someone to deal with my anus and feces than save the money and do it myself. That is, until I started getting really grumpy on Day 16. By Day 17, I had turned into the Grinch Who Stole Christmas and the Wicked Witch of the West combined. I could barely keep myself from snapping at everyone and saying every negative thing that came to mind. Over the course of two days, funky, nasty, mean thoughts that were completely unlike me bubbled up from God knows where. I was in such a bad mood, I knew to stay to myself before I said something mean that I'd later regret. I knew I was paying the price for not flushing the toxins out fast enough. I would have to give myself an enema or continue to be trapped in this cesspool of poisons and mean and nasty thoughts. On Day 19, I gave myself an enema, which was nowhere near as bad as I'd made it out to be. In fact, it wasn't uncomfortable at all. Immediately after doing the enema, I felt so much better. Until the caffeine really kicked in. It turns out that I'm caffeine sensitive. I stayed high on caffeine for 18 hours—I felt better but I was a mess! I ended my detox on Day 21, broke the detox correctly—which I found surprisingly easy; I thought I'd be ravished—then transitioned into maintenance eating, which was better than I've eaten in my entire life. I kept that up for four months, backslid somewhat, and am now getting back on the bandwagon. On what would have been the equivalent of Day 25 I got a colonic, and my hydrotherapist was stunned to see large, black, marble-sized balls of toxins come out of my body. We hadn't seen anything like that before and we haven't seen it since. After getting those toxins out of me, I felt better immediately.

A few days after the detox ended, I gave myself a pedicure. To my surprise, I noticed that there were far fewer spider veins on my ankle. I'd had spider veins as a teenager. I'd attributed them, in part, to spraining my ankles many times playing sports. Now, I realize that they reflected something unhealthy happening in my circulatory system— and that some of what was wrong had healed! I was also shocked to discover that I stopped needing deodorant—even in the 95-degree heat. (To be safe, I purchased a natural deodorant that didn't work on me before detoxing, but now works fine in all kinds of weather.) My internal thermostat changed as well. About a month after the detox, I traveled to New York on a sweltering, 100-plus-degree day. As I walked through the streets, I realized that I was hot but not wilting as everyone else was. I walked comfortably at my normal pace. I am no longer as hot on very hot days or as cold on cold days. My body seems not to be anywhere near as affected by the external temperature as it used to be—it's as though it regulates its thermostat better. My hair is growing incredibly quickly. And as for my fibroids? They seem smaller and something's definitely shifting about them. I no longer bloat before my period and the volume of my period has decreased by one-third. I intend to do the 7-day Detox yet again this year—who knows, I may keep going and make it to 21 days again!

9

ENDING THE DETOX

There is a story told in holistic circles about four women who attended a retreat to participate in a 21-day detox. Following the cleanse, they apparently were not told or did not "get" how important it was to come off their detox properly. Instead of gradually adding one food group at a time and avoiding foods laden with synthetic chemicals, they celebrated their success by going out for pizza and beer. Pizza is greasy and toxic with rancid, preservative-filled fats. Beer contains alcohol, which can be a poison or allergen, as well as toxic preservatives. All four of the women got sick. Two ended up in the hospital, one in anaphylactic shock, the most serious type of allergic reaction because it affects entire body systems including the respiratory tract and the cardiovascular system. Three of the women recovered, but the one in shock lost her life.

That reaction is a severe response to an extreme case. But I've had clients tell me they have experienced lesser reactions such as itching, scratchy throat, belching, nausea, and vomiting when they ate toxic foods too soon after a detox. You will experience reactions such as these only if you ignore the rules for breaking your detox.

Twenty-one days into the detox, you look and feel younger. Your body is lighter and more energetic. You feel better in your body. The cells in your body will be cleaner, lighter, and more open than they have been in many years. As long as you feed it healthy food, you will continue to look and feel vital and energetic.

But now that your body is clean, though it may have withstood processed and junk foods before you detoxed, it will no longer tolerate them afterwards. Every time you ingest toxic substances you will experience a noticeable physical reaction. Depending on how toxic the food is, your reaction may range from merely losing energy or feeling sleepy to burping or getting gassy or bloated, to itching or developing a rash, to getting a headache, to developing mild indigestion, to even becoming sick to your stomach. Returning to toxic eating habits will also cause you to gain weight, particularly if you do so immediately upon ending the detox, when your cells are clean and wide open. These reactions are a gift from your body, which now has the opportunity to teach you what foods it does or does not want to eat. My clients are shocked to discover just how poorly they had been treating themselves all along without knowing it. The fact that your body will react to toxic foods will make transitioning to a healthy diet much easier.

Awakening Your Digestive System

Whether you engage in a 21-day, 7-day, or weekend detox, it's very important to come off of your plan in a very specific manner that protects you from reintroducing too many toxins to your body too quickly, prevents you from regaining the weight you just lost, and helps you transition into eating habits that are healthier than you had before detoxing. Exactly how you break your fast depends upon the length of your detox. During this time you will awaken your digestive system gently by slowly adding all the food groups back into your diet, starting with a protein powder supplement and ending with animal protein. Protein plays an essential role in the body, from making enzymes to supporting the immune system. So you're going to get protein; just not in the form of meat. If you're a 21-day detoxer, I want you to drink one protein shake daily. Any flavor you want to drink is fine. If you detox for 7 days or a weekend, it is less important to resume protein immediately. Follow the instructions below for breaking those fasts. During this transitional period it will be important to eat modest amounts of food and not overeat. I'd like you to eat more slowly than you may be used to, taking the time to enjoy your food. I recommend chewing each bite a hundred times rather than scarfing it down, as we so often do because we spend so much time eating on the run. Also, pay attention to any reactions you may experience, such as indigestion, gas, constipation, diarrhea, or itchy skin, after eating certain foods, as you may uncover food intolerances or allergies you did not know you had.

Warning: DO NOT consume any alcoholic beverages, illegal drugs, cigarettes, or any other highly toxic substances for 11 days, if you do the 21-day detox; 4 days if you do the 7-day detox; or 1 day if you detox for 2 days. (The rule of thumb is: avoid noxious substances for half the number of days you detoxed.) You could land yourself in the hospital if you do not follow these rules. Here is a safe, day-by-day approach to breaking your fast.

Breaking the 21-day Detox

Day 1

Continue consuming your juice, cleansing soups, broth, and all of your supplements. By now, you may be craving protein. Add one protein shake today. For lunch, eat a very small cup of raw vegetable salad or cooked vegetable with no dressing, oil, or vinegar.

Day 2

Continue eating the foods and supplements you ate on Day 1. You may also eat a small cup of fruit as long as you eat it two hours away from meals.

Day 3

Repeat Day 2, adding one serving of a whole-grain cereal like oatmeal, whole wheat, or brown rice.

Day 4

Repeat Day 3, adding an essential fatty acid liquid or flaxseed oil. For example, try one teaspoon of flaxseed oil or an essential fatty acid liquid or capsules with a salad, vegetable dish, or a protein drink.

Day 5

Repeat Day 4, adding other proteins such as eggs, soy, nuts, legumes, and beans (pinto beans, black-eyed peas, and/or kidney beans).

Day 6

You may now add three to four ounces of boiled, broiled, or baked fish and chicken to your diet. Try not to consume animal protein more then three times per week. Continue to drink protein smoothies or rice-and-bean dishes on the days that you are not consuming meat.

Day 7

If you wish, you may add red meat to the list of foods you ate on Day 6.

After breaking your fast by completing Day 7, you now transition into your maintenance diet, a wholesome diet that is ideally synthetic-chemical free but at least should contain far fewer toxins than you were eating in the past. You will continue to lose weight while on the maintenance program. Follow these maintenance principles:

- Cook and serve foods in healthy ways.
- Continue drinking plenty of water, drinking your supplements, and using enzymes.
- Take one enzyme with each chewing meal to assist with digestion.

- Consume one protein shake on days you are not consuming animal products.
- Eat one serving of non-fat organic yogurt with live cultures to add friendly bacteria to your system.
- As you transition back into your life, make a point of engaging in at least one weekly detox treatment, such as getting a colonic or massage, brushing your skin, or taking a detox bath, to continue to rid your body of new toxins.

Days 8–11 Are Examples of Maintenance Days

Day 8

Breakfast: One 8-ounce glass/bottle of water, antioxidant berry drink; one enzyme capsule; oatmeal with cinnamon, nutmeg, or organic vanilla flavoring. You may add rice, almond, or soy milk.

Snack: One 8-ounce glass/bottle of water (green drink).

Lunch: One enzyme capsule, one 8-ounce glass/bottle of water. Steamed vegetables on plate of mixed greens (make your own salad dressing).

Snack: Protein shake (you may add liquid essential fatty acid or flaxseed oils); one 8-ounce glass/bottle of water.

Dinner: One enzyme capsule, three to four ounces of salmon on a plate of spinach.

Snack: One 8-ounce cup of hot or iced herbal tea (it's okay to add lemon and stevia); one cup of plain non-fat organic yogurt with live cultures (you may add essential fats, or organic flavorings, like vanilla extract).

Day 9

Breakfast: One 8-ounce glass/bottle of water with antioxidant berry drink; one enzyme capsule; egg omelet (made with

two eggs) with chopped onions, mushrooms, chopped broccoli, or your favorite vegetables. Use olive oil lightly or essential fatty acids that contain omega 3 and 6.

Snack: One 8-ounce glass/bottle green drink.

Lunch: One enzyme capsule, three to four ounces of broiled
or baked chopped chicken, chopped garlic, green pepper,
onions, and seasoning dressing. You can make your own dressing with oil, balsamic vinegar, or Bragg's amino acid. Wrap
with large pieces of greens, lettuce, or protein bread.

Snack: Green drink; one 8-ounce glass/bottle of water.

Dinner: One enzyme capsule, vegetable cleansing soups
(make fresh soup with lots of green vegetables garlic and
onions). Add brown rice.

Snack: One 8-ounce cup of hot or iced herbal tea (lemon and
stevia can be added); one cup of plain non-fat organic yogurt
with live cultures (you may add nuts, essential fats, or organic
flavorings, like vanilla extract).

Day 10

Breakfast: One cup of mixed fruit of your choice; one enzyme
capsule.

Snack: One 8-ounce glass/bottle of water with antioxidant
berry drink; if your berry drink is liquid rather than powdered,
you may drink it without the water.

Lunch: One enzyme capsule; one cup of brown rice with one
cup of spicy beans (see recipe on p. 208).

Snack: One 8-ounce glass/bottle of water with added green
drink formula.

Dinner: One enzyme capsule; one cup of stir-fried curry
vegetables; and one protein shake *or* three to four ounces of
chicken or fish.

Snack: One 8-ounce cup of hot or iced herbal tea (lemon and stevia can be added); one cup of plain non-fat organic yogurt with live cultures (you may add essential fats, or organic flavorings, like vanilla extract).

Day 11

Breakfast: One 8-ounce glass/bottle of water with protein shake (you may add essential fatty acid liquid or flaxseed oil); one enzyme capsule; one cup of natural granola with rice or almond milk (no dairy).

Snack: One 8-ounce glass/bottle of water with antioxidant berry drink; if your berry drink is liquid rather than powdered, you may drink it without the water.

Lunch: Three to four ounces of tuna salad over a bed of greens; one enzyme capsule.

Snack: Green drink/bottle of water.

Dinner: One enzyme capsule; one cup of spicy tofu with one cup of mixed vegetables.

Snack: One 8-ounce cup of hot or iced herbal tea (lemon and stevia can be added); one cup plain non-fat organic yogurt with live cultures (you may add essential fats, or organic flavorings, like vanilla extract).

Breaking the 7-day Detox

When breaking a weeklong fast, follow these instructions:

Day 1

Continue consuming your juice, cleansing soups, broth and all of your supplements. You may also eat a small cup of fruit, as long as you eat it two hours away from meals. For lunch, eat a very small cup of raw vegetable salad or cooked vegetable with no dressing, oil, or vinegar.

Day 2

Continue eating the foods and supplements you ate on Day 1, adding one serving of a whole-grain cereal like oatmeal, whole wheat, or brown rice.

Day 3

Repeat Day 2, adding an essential fatty acid liquid or flaxseed oil. For example, add one teaspoon of flaxseed oil or an essential fatty acid liquid to a salad or vegetable dish. Today, you can also add protein to your diet in the form of protein powder. For example, try making a protein smoothie, adding flaxseed oil or an essential fatty acid liquid to it.

Day 4

Repeat Day 3, adding other proteins such as eggs, soy, nuts, legumes and beans. You may now add 3–4 ounces of boiled, broiled, or baked fish and chicken to your diet. I recommend selecting organic. You may add red meat the next day if you wish.

Breaking the 2-day Detox

When breaking a weekend fast, follow these instructions:

Day 1

Continue consuming your juice, cleansing soups, broth, and all of your supplements. You must be careful today to eat only healthy foods without chemicals and toxins. I recommend that you chew well, stay hydrated, and move your bowels daily. Tomorrow, you may begin the maintenance program below. I suggest following it until you detox again.

Whether you are breaking the 21-day, 7-day, or 2-day detox, it is important that you continue drinking six to eight ounces of water between meals, totaling forty-eight to sixty-four ounces daily.

What Should I Eat Now? The Maintenance Program

Now that you've invested in losing weight and cleaning up your body, doesn't it make sense to keep it healthy? Who wants to go back to living in a body that was heavy and felt lousy? Instead, why not use this opportunity to build upon the good habits and feelings you've developed over the past three weeks, using the detox as the catalyst to help you create a healthier, lighter-weight lifestyle? I recommend that you keep exercising daily, using the maintenance menus from Days 8 through 11 as examples of healthy eating, and follow these healthy-eating guidelines and schedule repeated detox. Now that you've completed one, it will be easier to do another. I suggest that you engage in one 21-day detox once a year, a 7-day cleanup each calendar season, or a weekend detox each week.

Eat More

- Eat a balanced diet containing nutrients from each food group—protein, fruit, vegetables, grains, healthy fats, vitamins, and minerals, following the food-combining concepts below.
- Focus on eating natural foods since the body recognizes and metabolizes them more easily, helping you avoid digestive discomforts and maintain your lighter weight.
- Eat as many whole foods in their natural state as possible; for example, unprocessed brown or wild rice instead of white; old-fashioned, instead of instant or flavored, oatmeal; whole-grain cereal instead of processed or presweetened; fresh fruit and vegetables instead of juice drinks or fruit roll-ups.
- One-half to three-fourths of your diet should be comprised of living foods, like fresh fruits and vegetables, where the enzymes are alive.
- Consume maximum nutritional supplements in small doses. Examples: green drinks, antioxidant berry drink, and protein shakes.

Make Salad Dressings

As you incorporate more salads and fresh vegetables into your diet, there's no need to weigh them down with toxin-laden toppings. Why not use your blender and food processor to create wonderful homemade salad dressings instead? For instance, try mixing Bragg's amino acids with ginger; or cucumbers, celery, tomatoes, yogurt, parsley, and herbal seasoning; or creole seasoning and balsamic vinaigrette. If you want a thicker dressing, put the ingredients in the blender. If you want a more fluid dressing, juice the vegetable ingredients. The combinations are as limitless as your imagination—or you can read the natural ingredients on the back of your favorite commercial salad dressing and improvise from there, without preservatives, of course. Each dressing takes only five to ten minutes to make and you have enough for a few days. And once you taste how wonderful freshly made dressings taste, you may never go back to the store-bought brands.

Healthy homemade salad-dressing ingredients:
- Bragg's amino acids
- Balsamic vinegar
- Rice vinegar
- Ginger
- Onion
- Lemon
- Lime
- Garlic
- Hot sauce
- Fresh herbs, spices, and/or salt-free seasonings

Add to Your Diet:

- **Nonmeat protein.** To avoid consuming excessive amounts of saturated fat, I suggest eating animal products, particularly chicken and fish but no red meat, no more than two times per week; eat rice and beans once or twice weekly; and one protein shake three to four times weekly.
- **Probiotics.** By adding good or "friendly" bacteria to the intestinal tract we can help our body digest food more effectively, strengthen our immune system to resist diseases, and regulate and maintain our health and vitality. One way to do this is by eating yogurt that contains at least 10 billion

cultures of probiotics. I recommend adding essential fats, or organic flavorings like vanilla extract. I do not like yogurt with added fruit since fruit digests best when eaten alone (see food-combining concepts below). You can have one serving of yogurt per day, preferably after dinner. If you don't like yogurt, take probiotic supplements. But I'll be perfectly honest with you: all the probiotics in the world can't help you if your eating habits are awful and/or your colon health is bad. If you go back to the standard American diet, the benefits of probiotics will be short lived.

- **Fiber.** Also known as roughage or bulk, fiber is best known for its ability to increase the weight and size of your stool

---

Six Rules for Food Combining

You can avoid common digestive problems like gas, bloating, and acid indigestion, by following these guidelines for combing your food:

1. Eat protein with vegetables only. Protein digests easier when you consume it with veggies.
2. Eat starches—like rice, grains, bread, potatoes, pasta, flour—with vegetables only. Starches digest easier with veggies. So when you eat a sandwich, in addition to using whole-grain bread, add foods like lettuce, tomato, or avocado.
3. Eat fruit by itself, two hours before or after meals. The enzymes in fruit digest better if you eat them alone, which makes fruit the perfect food to snack on.
4. Eat rice and beans together. Almost anywhere you travel in the world, you will find some indigenous meal comprised of rice and beans. Together, they form a complete protein, containing all of the essential amino acids. You can substitute this for animal protein.
5. Eat omega-3 and omega-6 oils with protein. It is hard for the body to digest protein alone; the body digests it better in combination with omega oils. You can eat fish like salmon, sardines, or mackerel, which are high in these oils. Or you can purchase liquid essential fatty acids, 3-6-9 oil, or flaxseed oil from the health-food store, then combine one teaspoon into a protein shake.
6. Eat animal sources of protein no more than three times per week. Animal protein is full of artery-clogging saturated fat. Instead, eat more protein from vegetable sources, rice, beans, and nuts, which are lighter, and contain good essential fatty acid liquid or flaxseed oils and don't clog your veins.

while softening it, thus preventing and easing constipation. It lowers the risk of diabetes and heart disease, but it may also aid weight loss and weight management, since high-fiber foods take longer to chew, giving the body more time to figure out that you're full, and thus making it less likely that you'll overeat. Fiber is classified into two categories—soluble and insoluble—based on whether it does (soluble) or does not (insoluble) dissolve in water. The body needs both. So eat a wide variety of high-fiber foods, such as whole wheat, wheat germ, nuts, oats, peas, beans, apples, citrus fruits, carrots, barley, and psyllium.

- **Essential fatty acid (EFA) liquid or flaxseed oils.** These are fats that the body cannot make on its own so we must obtain them from our diet. EFA deficiency is common in the United States—particularly omega-3 deficiency—contributing to many serious health conditions, including obesity, heart attacks, stroke, cancer, insulin resistance, diabetes, depression, asthma, lupus, and attention deficit hyperactivity disorder (ADHD). Add it to your diet by eating salmon (omega-3), whole grains, nuts, and seeds (omega-6), olive oil (omega-9), or a salad oil containing the three in combination, such as omega 3-6-9.

Eat Fewer

- Foods containing artificial flavors, colors, preservatives, pesticides, hormones, and antibiotics.
- Unnatural sugars like sucrose, fructose, maltodextrine, and the sugar substitutes in the yellow, pink, and blue packages.
- Do not add salt to your food. Eat only foods that contain natural sources of sodium, such as celery and kelp.
- Try getting your calcium from fruit, vegetables, and fish, instead. You may also use a calcium supplement. The American Dietary Association recommends that women get at least 1,200–1,500 mg of calcium a day and men should get about 1,000–1,200 mg.

Shop Smarter

- Shop the perimeter of the store, where the fresh foods are sold and there are fewer processed items
- Avoid the prepared foods department, where fried foods like chicken abound and ingredients like butter, whole milk, trans fats, salt, sugar, and artificial flavors are often used to make foods look, smell, and taste better.
- Read the labels of any prepared or processed foods you buy, minimizing the number of ingredients whose names you can't pronounce, look like chemicals, or you don't recognize as a food.

RECIPES

SOUPS

Many people on the Diet Detox take comfort in making their favorite soup; others prefer to be creative and concoct their own healthy vegetable blend. It doesn't matter which approach you take—as long as you exclude salt, sugar, milk/cream, eggs, butter, and alcohol (that includes wine). Below, you'll find recipes for some of my favorite blends. Their flavors come from around the world, so your taste buds won't get bored.

Asian Spinach Soup

Makes 2 servings

1 quart distilled water
2 cloves fresh garlic
1 tablespoon Bragg's liquid amino acids
¼ inch piece fresh ginger, peeled and chopped
3 cups fresh spinach, chopped
1 cup any other greens
½ cup green beans, chopped
1 teaspoon Asian chili sauce

Combine water, garlic, Bragg's, and fresh ginger in a large saucepan. Add cut-up vegetables. Boil over high heat until tender. Pour roughly ¼ cup of broth into a blender (add more for thicker soup), along with all of the vegetables and chili sauce. Puree and eat the soup. Drink the remaining broth.

Southern Collard Greens

Makes 2 servings

1 quart distilled water
3 cups fresh collards, chopped
½ cup green beans, chopped
½ cup carrots, peeled and chopped
1 stalk celery, chopped
4 cloves garlic, chopped
1 tablespoon no-salt seasoning
2 pinches cayenne pepper
1 pinch paprika
1 tablespoon fresh parsley, chopped

Add cut-up vegetables and spices to the water in a large saucepan. Boil over high heat until tender enough to blend. Puree and eat the soup. Drink the remaining broth.

Curried Vegetables

Makes 2 servings

1 quart water
1 cup carrots, chopped
1 cup mixed greens, chopped
1 cup yellow zucchini, chopped
1 cup green beans, chopped
1 green onion, chopped
4 cloves garlic, chopped
1 teaspoon curry powder
1 teaspoon turmeric powder
1 teaspoon mixture of ground cinnamon, nutmeg, ginger, and cayenne powder

Pour water into saucepan. Add all other ingredients, including spices, and boil until vegetables are tender over high heat. Taste the broth. If you find it too spicy, add more water. Next, pour approximately ¼ cup of broth into a blender, along with all of the vegetables. Puree and eat the soup. Drink the remaining broth.

Creamy Broccoli

Makes 2 servings

1 quart distilled water
Oregano, to taste
1 cup cauliflower, chopped
Flat-leaf parsley, to taste
Garlic, to taste
2 cups broccoli, chopped
1 cup green beans, chopped
1 cup carrots, peeled and chopped

Boil cauliflower, oregano, parsley, and garlic in 2 cups of water over high heat until completely soft. Blend until creamy, then set aside. In 4 cups of water, boil broccoli, green beans, and carrots, along with a dash of your favorite spice or no-salt seasoning, until all vegetables are soft enough to blend. Pour ⅛ cup of broth into blender and add softened vegetables. Blend to a thick consistency. Add the cauliflower cream on top.

Ginger Carrots

Makes 2 servings

1 quart distilled water
1 cup carrots, peeled and chopped
1 cup mixed greens
½ cup sweet potatoes, peeled and chopped
¼ inch piece ginger root, peeled and chopped
1 teaspoon mixture ground cinnamon, gloves, nutmeg, and stevia, to taste
1 teaspoon organic vanilla extract

Boil all vegetables with spices over high heat and blend. Next, pour ¼ cup of broth into a blender, along with all of the vegetables. Add vanilla extract at the end for taste. Puree and eat the soup. Drink the remaining broth.

Italian Green Beans

Makes 2 servings

1 quart water
2 cups green beans, chopped
1 cup mixed greens, spinach, collards, or kale
½ cup carrots, peeled and chopped
1 stalk celery, chopped
4 cloves garlic, chopped
¼ teaspoon cayenne pepper
1 tablespoon mixture chopped fresh oregano, basil, rosemary, and flat-leaf parsley
1 bay leaf

Boil all vegetables in a large saucepan over high heat, blend, and drink the broth. If broth is too spicy, add water. Next, pour approximately ¼ of broth into a blender, along with all of the vegetables. Puree and eat the soup. Drink the remaining broth.

Spicy Beans

Makes 2 servings

1 quart water
1½ cups black beans
3 pinches thyme
1 onion, diced
¼ clove of garlic
1 pinch cayenne pepper
1 teaspoon tomato paste
1 teaspoon no-salt vegetable seasoning

Place all of the ingredients in a medium-sized saucepan. Cook on medium heat for approximately 45 minutes or until the beans are nice and tender.

DR. RONI'S FAVORITE SALAD DRESSINGS

Why buy healthy and perhaps even organic vegetables only to weigh them down with commercially prepared salad dressings that are laden with toxins? Healthy, homemade salad dressings taste fresh, are easy to make, and spare you the chemical chaser. You can also add these seasoning blends to vegetable soup for additional flavor.

Do not use these recipes while you're detoxing; they're for when you're on a maintenance plan.

Italian Naturally Dressing

1 pinch minced garlic
1 pinch basil
1 pinch oregano
1 pinch parsley
1 pinch cayenne
1 tablespoon no-salt vegetable seasoning
½ cup balsamic vinegar
1 tablespoon essential fatty acid

Puree all ingredients in a blender until smooth. Chill before serving.

Cucumber Onion Dressing

2 tablespoons red onion, finely chopped
2 tablespoons cucumber, finely chopped
Pinch basil, chopped
¼ teaspoon vegetable seasoning
¼ teaspoon garlic powder
Pinch cayenne pepper
¼ cup of red wine vinegar
½ teaspoon of essential fatty acid

Puree all ingredients in a blender until smooth. Chill before serving.

Spicy Green Bean Vinaigrette Dressing

¼ cup fresh lemon juice
¼ cup rice vinegar
1 handful green beans
1 pinch garlic powder
1 pinch cayenne pepper

Puree all ingredients in a blender until smooth. For thicker or thinner dressing, increase or reduce amount of green beans. Chill before serving.

Spicy Mustard Dressing

¼ teaspoon Bragg's liquid amino acid
2 tablespoons spicy rice vinegar
2 teaspoons organic mustard
Plain nonfat yogurt to taste
1 pinch stevia

To Bragg's, rice vinegar, and mustard, add yogurt until creamy to your likeness; add stevia to taste. Chill before serving.

Sweet & Sour Carrot Dressing

¼ cup red wine vinegar
¼ cup carrot juice
¼ cup tomatoes, mashed
1 teaspoon lemon juice
1 pinch paprika
2 packs stevia

Puree all ingredients in a blender until smooth. Chill before serving.

DAILY SALAD

Enjoy any variety of organic green salad with mixed vegetables daily. This is one of my favorites.

Vegetable Chunk Salad

Makes 2 servings

1 large red or green bell pepper, chopped into bite-size pieces
½ red onion, diced
½ cucumber, chopped into bite-size pieces
2 celery stalks, chopped into small pieces
10 to 12 cherry tomatoes, halved
½ yellow squash, chopped into bite-size pieces
3 to 4 tablespoons of your favorite essential fatty acid
3 tablespoons red wine vinegar
¼ teaspoon powdered stevia
1 teaspoon dried Italian seasoning
1 pinch cayenne pepper
2 tablespoons Braggs Amino Acid

Place all the chopped vegetables in a medium-sized bowl. Place the essential fatty acid, vinegar, stevia, Italian seasoning, cayenne pepper, and the Braggs Amino Acid in a small plastic container with a lid. Close lid and shake dressing vigorously for 1 minute. Pour dressing over salad and toss.

WEIGHT-MAINTENANCE SHAKES

Not everyone who wants to detox their body also wants to lose weight. If you're one of the lucky few folks who don't struggle with size, you'll have to take some extra steps to keep from shedding pounds. Martha's Vineyard Holistic Retreat naturopath Linda Hicks has plenty of experience caring for elderly patients whose appetites were poor yet needed to maintain their weight. She has developed these recipes for high-calorie shakes that contain no animal ingredients.

Orange-Cream Frappe

2 scoops vanilla protein powder

1 scoop orange-flavored natural fiber

1 drop pure orange oil or orange flavor extract

2 ounces distilled water

6 ounces coconut milk, Rice Dream, soy milk, or almond milk

Mix all ingredients in blender and whip at maximum speed until ice-cream consistency. More liquid may be added to the recipe to improve its "drinkability," but eating it with a spoon makes it seem like a thick dessert.

Yam Surprise

2 scoops vanilla protein powder

1 small baking or sweet potato, peeled

1 packet stevia

½ teaspoon organic vanilla

3 ounces distilled water

5 ounces of organic coconut milk, almond milk, soy milk, or rice milk

1 teaspoon essential fatty acid, only if you use soy milk, almond milk, or rice milk

6 ice cubes

1 teaspoon ground nutmeg

Mix all ingredients in blender and whip at maximum speed until ice-cream consistency. Pour into a glass and sprinkle nutmeg on top.

GLOSSARY

Acidic: A chemical compound that yields a solution with a pH of less than 7 when dissolved in water.

Acidophilus: "Good bacteria" found in yogurts.

Alkaline: Having a pH of between 7 and 14.

Allergic reaction: The body's response when it cannot tolerant something foreign. Also referred to as hypersensitivity.

Amino acid: A component of proteins, which contain various proportions of about twenty common amino acids.

Antibiotic: Medicine that prevents and treats infectious diseases.

Antihypertensive medication: Medicine that helps lower blood pressure.

Antioxidant: A chemical that slows or halts oxidation, the rusting of the body.

Bacteria: A major group of living organisms. Depending on the type, bacteria can be either good or bad for the body.

Body mass index (BMI): Defined as one's body weight divided by the square of their height (weight/height^2). Your BMI measures whether you weigh too much or too little.

Bowel movement: The process by which the body eliminates waste in the form of feces.

Calorie: Energy we get from food.

Cancer: A malignant and invasive growth or tumor.

Carbon dioxide: A colorless, odorless, incombustible gas often abbreviated as CO_2.

Cascara sagrada: Dried aged bark of a small tree in the buckthorn family native to the Pacific Northwest.

Catalyze: To modify or bring about.

Central nervous system: Regulates all motor and sensory activity in our body.

Chi machine: A machine that stimulates the lymphatic system by swinging your lower extremities while you lie down with your feet in the machine.

Cholesterol: Fat that builds up in the arteries and contributes to development of heart disease.

Chronically ill: Having an illness that lasts for a long time.

Colon: The primary organ that eliminates waste and toxins from the body. When the colon is clean, the body is able to purify itself more easily.

Colon hydrotherapy: Similar to an enema but using a machine, a colonic introduces large amounts of purified water into the colon in order to cleanse it.

Degenerative disease: A disease that slowly destroys one or more organs.

Denature: To deprive of its natural qualities or change the nature of.

Detoxify: To rid the body of poison or the effect of poison.

Diabetes: A chronic disease that occurs when the body produces or uses too little insulin and causes excessive amounts of glucose to appear in the blood and urine.

Dietary deficiency: Occurs when the body does not receive enough nutrients.

Endocrine system: Controls our hormones.

Enema: A method of introducing water, herbs, coffee, or other active agents into the colon to soften fecal sludge and impacted stools.

Enzyme: A protein that causes or speeds up the body's various chemical reactions. For instance, digestive enzymes are needed for proper digestion to occur.

Equilibrium: A state of balance.

Fat (body): The fat contained in your body.

Fat (dietary): Fat obtained from one's diet. Dietary fat offers nine calories per gram.

Fatty essential acids: Fatty acids required by the human body but which the body cannot make so must be acquired through the diet.

Free radical: An atom or group of atoms with at least one unpaired electron. In the body it is usually an oxygen molecule that has lost an electron and will stabilize itself by stealing an electron from a nearby molecule, causing oxidation.

Germ: A good or bad bacterium, also referred to as a pathogen.

Glycogen: The principal form in which the body stores glucose (sugar).

Heart disease: An abnormality in the heart's structure or function, or of the blood vessels supplying the heart, that keeps the heart from functioning normally.

Herbicide: A chemical substance used to destroy or inhibit the growth of plants, particularly weeds.

High-density lipoprotein (HDL) cholesterol: Also known as "good" cholesterol, high HDL levels are associated with a decreased risk of atherosclerosis and coronary heart disease.

High-density nutritional supplements: A small dose of nutrients containing extra and higher-quality nutrition

Homeostasis: A state of being in harmony and balance.

Hormones: Chemicals manufactured by the endocrine system to help control many bodily functions.

Immune system: A specialized system of cells and organs that protects our body from negative outside biological influences.

Inflammation: The immune system's first response to infection or irritation.

Litmus paper: Filter paper impregnated with water-soluble dye. Used as a pH indicator to test materials for acidity.

Low-density lipoprotein (LDL) cholesterol: Also known as "bad" cholesterol, high levels of LDL cholesterol increase one's risk of atherosclerosis and coronary heart disease.

Lycopene: A red pigment found in blood and tomatoes, which is a potent antioxidant.

Lymph-drainage massage: A gentle form of massage incorporating a gentle pumping action to stimulate the lymphatic system.

Lymph nodes: Act as a biological filter cleaning out microorganisms from fluids.

Malnutrition: Occurs when the body does not receive enough nutrients.

Metabolic rate: The speed with which your body burns up calories.

Metabolism: The rate at which your body burns food.

Minerals: Elements our body needs to keep us healthy. Examples include copper, silver, and magnesium.

Molecules: Smallest particle of a substance.

Nicotine: A toxic yet addictive chemical released from cigarette smoke.

Noxious: Hurtful or harmful.

Nutrient: Any element or compound necessary for or contributing to an organism's metabolism, growth, or other function.

Nutritional detox: A process of stimulating the body to rid itself of bad nutrition and replace it with higher quality.

Omega-3: An essential fatty acid found in the oil of vegetables and oily fish.

Organic: All natural and containing no synthetic ingredients.

Oxidation: A chemical reaction that occurs when a substance combines with oxygen.

Oxygen: A molecule that helps carry red blood cells throughout our body and is essential to survival.

Parasite cleanse: A detox that expels parasites from the intestinal system.

Peristalsis: The wavelike muscular contractions of the alimentary canal or other tubular structures by which contents are forced onward toward the opening.

Pesticide: A chemical used to kill pests, especially insects.

Probiotics: Good bacteria called flora found mostly in the digestive tract.

Protein: An essential component of our diet found in meats, eggs, beans, vegetables, and dairy products and that the body needs for energy.

Purge: To rid of impurities.

Rebounder: A small trampoline that stimulates and assists the lymphatic system.

Sedentary: Accustomed to sitting or engaging in little exercise.

Sick soil: Soil lacking in vital nutrients.

Synthetic: Man-made.

Toxic burden/toxic load: The level of pollutants, poisonous or harmful substances carried around in the body.

Toxin: A poisonous substance capable of producing disease.

Virus: A parasitic particle that is so small that it's invisible to the naked eye, but that infects cells in biological organisms.

Vitamins: Water-soluble and fat-soluble nutrients that feed the body and keep it healthy.

White-coat hypertension: Occurs when a person's blood pressure rises when they see a medical professional wearing the white coat often worn by health care providers.

Yeast: A type of fungus that is found in one's body.

ACKNOWLEDGMENTS

RONI DELUZ

First, I offer all of my love and appreciation to God, for He has brought this life and all of you to me. I give my thanks to my family. Mom and Dad, you are always there and your love has never faltered. Grandma, I blossomed in the light you shined upon me. Antonio DeLuz, father of my children and lifetime partner, you have been patient and giving throughout all of my life's endeavors. Whitney, Toron, and Tony Jr., you are my angels. Jamie and James, I am so grateful I have you to help me with the children while I am on the road. Carol, Lenore, and James, my precious siblings, I appreciate your prayers and love. Kathy and Lorraine, you provide me with a constant flow of love.

So many people have lighted the way, leading me to my present life, that it's hard to know where to begin. Deborah Williams, green juice, those "crazy" treatments and all, thank you for persisting and putting me on the path. Thank you also for introducing me to James Hester.

James, my life has moved at warp speed ever since I met you. You challenged me to write this book. I'll always be grateful to you for telling me that if I didn't feel inclined to write it for myself that I should do it for others. Back then I thought it would never happen, but you made me a believer. We did it! I am honored to have you as my business partner. You taught me about believing in the dream of helping millions of people through books and education. I taught you about health and wellness. . . . The world will be better off because you took this risk and I congratulate you for your courage. I am proud to say I watched you grow mentally, physically, and spiritually, and I know the world will embrace you as we join in this journey of helping people change their lives. Everyone should have a James Hester in their lives—I'm blessed to have one.

Thanks also to the following people: Susan Swartz, for your unique, creative essence and support of the retreat in so many ways; Linda Hicks, for your commitment and all the wisdom you share at the retreat; Pamela Ray, my lifelong friend who has been with me from the beginning; Cathy Hughes, for having faith in me and my cause; Jaime Foster Brown and Lorenzo Brown, you are true believers and you have helped so many; Dr. Douglas Rofrano, I won't forget you for always lending your spiritual wit. My pastor, Marcia Buckley, you are forever giving. Hilary Beard, for fashioning my voice into words for all who will listen; Judith Regan, there are no words to express my gratitude; Laurye Blackford, for your wonderful editor's eye. Thank you, John Rose, in the last hour of need. Thank you, Dr. Nicholas, for many medical and spiritual talks; Dr. Lorna Andrade, for being there in the beginning and for our long-term friendship; Heather Rynd, for your positive energy; and Lauren Horten, for your friendship and sharing. Lisa Adler—you changed me. Dr. Monica Turner—thanks for the healthy knowledge. And many others. There are many others—special clients, friends, and angels—who have helped me create my dream.

Thank you all,

Roni DeLuz, RN, ND, PhD
Vineyard Haven, Martha's Vineyard, Massachusetts

JAMES HESTER

I would like to give all praise and glory to God for leading me to Martha's Vineyard. I heard him speak to me on my third day at Dr. Roni's retreat. The voice said, "Do my will and pass the healing on to those in need." He also led me to Pastor Marcia Buckley on Easter Sunday 2003. My life has been changed ever since. I love and thank these two amazing women.

I would like to thank all of those who allowed me to pass the gift God gave me unto them. I pray that they will pass the gift on to their family, friends, and colleagues. When a loved one is in their darkest hour, we have the power to make their days brighter. Here are a few that made my days brighter:

My father (Jim Hester), my mother (Loretta Hester), my sisters (Judi Thompson and Michelle Alfo), my aunts (Joan Walsh and Geri Trzanowski). Bethann Hardison, my dear friend, adviser, and confidant. Judith Regan, thank you for allowing us into your world and believing in this project. Cathy Hughes, thanks for your love and support. I love you all very much. I'm so proud of you all giving your bodies the gift of detoxing.

My lifelong friends: Butch and Regina Woolfolk, Donna Fuime, David Cole, Lucy Doughty, Dr. Judy Meyers, Robert Evans, Maye James, Lorainne Van Rensailer, Gina Franano, Timolin Cole, Al Zelenka, Tommy Thompson, and Sondra "Miss Everything" Fortunato. You all have your own stories about me and I thank and love you for always letting James be James.

My healing team: Dr. Roni DeLuz, Dr. Martinez, Dr. L. Miller, Dr. Michael Hickson, Dr. Gervais Frechette, Evelyn "Diva" Harrington, Ene Luna and Laura Rios (Juarez, Mexico). My angels at the retreat, Pamela Ray (the best colon therapist in the world) and Linda Hicks (I love you both so much and I'm very grateful that you are in my life), Linda Gonzalez, Celina Pina, and Deborah Williams. Mr. and Mrs. Oxygen—Ed and Leeda McCabe—thanks for educating me about Ozone. Maria Alonzo (NY) and Jason Peringer (Martha's Vineyard), my massage therapists. These are some of the most gifted professional in their fields. Thank you for caring and healing.

Mariah Carey, thank you for sending our "sister" Deborah Cooper to Dr. Roni. You saved her life—you're an angel. Also, Barbara and Andrew Pace, Melonie Daniels, and Michael Richardson—for hearing the 911 call and responding immediately. Thanks for caring. God bless you.

Brad Boles, Anne Austin, Jackie Malloy, Alvaro, Marvet Britto, Tyrone Barrington, Paris Gordon, and Judy Moskowitz, thanks for standing and listening to me as I told the truth. . . . The truth will set you free . . .

Robin Quivers thank you for allowing us into your home and life—you are changing people's lives—we thank you for the opportunity of detoxing you every day on *The Howard Stern Radio Show*. We would also like to thank Howard Stern, Artie Lange, Fred Norris, Gary Dell'Abate, Ronnie and Tim Sabean for protecting, supporting, and believing in Dr. Roni and allowing her to educate your listeners regarding their health . . . Larry King, Bill Geddie, and Mercedes Torres—thanks for the support . . .

Wendy Williams at 107.5: we had a blast detoxing you every day live on the radio. Joannetta "Supermom" Patton: we had a blast detoxing you in Atlanta. Joanna Yearwood: you look great. Oscar Hernandez: we have to detox again. Rosalie Forest—our first at home graduate.

Some of the most anointed singers, producers, and executives in the music business blessed me with the opportunity and privilege of working with them. Here are just a few I would like to thank: Natalie Cole ("Livin' for Love"), thank you for bringing me to church—you planted the seed. Mary J. Blige/Aretha Franklin ("Don't Waste Your Time")—Mary, you are correct, there are lessons in the valley. Marc Anthony ("Remember Me"), how's Bigram? Kelly Price/Teddy Reilly ("Love Sets You Free")—TR, you're a musical genius. Jeff Majors ("Pray"), the most gifted composer and harpist in the world. Billy Porter—what a voice. Robert Clivilles (C&C Music Factory), you are so talented. Dj Hex Hector ("This is My Moment to Shine"), DJ Father Chris and

DJ Sin, and the best DJ in the world, Erick Morillo—thanks for being my friend . . . your 21 days is coming . . . Three of the most talented music executives: Sylvia Rhone, Clive Davis, and Antonio "LA" Reid. Gen Rubin—you are so talented—we made hits together! Randy "American Idol" Jackson, I'm so proud of your new career—you deserve it. Alfred Liggins (Radio One)—thanks for being a friend and sharing Cathy with me. My Three Divas: Deborah Cooper, Melonie Daniels, and MaryAnn Tatum—these girls can *sing*. We had a lot of fun. Three gentlemen that left us too soon: David Cole—my brother and friend—what a talent, there is no other. Frankie Crocker—thanks for the break at age 14—what an ear. Luther Vandross—thanks for allowing me to work with you on "You Really Started Something." What an honor. May you rest in peace. May God continue to bless all of you and thanks again for the opportunity. If you ever need to get healthy—I'm one call away. It continues to be a personal and spiritual growth, a process that led me to this book.

Maureen Orth, Jamie Foster Brown, Mitch Albom, Bob Adams, Richard Johnson and Paula Froelich (Page Six), George Rush and Joanna Molloy, and Jancee Dunn (*Vogue*)—the first journalists to write about us. Plum TV of Martha's Vineyard (Stephon, Kelly, John, and Guinevere). John Meade and all the saints at the Martha's Vineyard Apostolic House of Prayer. Bishop Philip Campbell. Pastor A.R. Bernard (CCC) for giving me a home away from home in NY. Thank you all for your support.

Alison Leopold (next one), Lynne Johnson, Jaime Rua, Barbara Burns, John Rose, thanks for all your legal advise.

Hilary Beard—you are such a talented writer.

Jaime Camil—another angel sent from God—I love you very much for helping to save my life.

I would like to thank the entire Hester, Darata, Mickiewicz, Kot, Trzanowski, Walsh, Ehlers, Thompson, and Zelenka families for their prayers and support. Your family will always be there for you.

Thank you to all the praying people in the world. Prayer is powerful.

This book is dedicated to my favorite boys: My nephews Cole and Kyle Thompson, Jarrel and Troy Woolfolk, and Sean and Lucas Doughty. If you take care of your body, your body will take care of you. The lessons you learn in the valley are just as important and valuable as the lessons you learn on top of the peak. Remember always to put God and your wonderful parents first in your life.

Man's rejection is God's protection.

James Hester
Martha's Vineyard

Dear Wellness Friend,

Congratulations and I'm proud of you for taking the step toward a healthier new you.

Please visit **www.mvdietdetox.com** *for updated information on:*

- *Helpful suggestions*
- *New schedules and changes*
- *New recipes*
- *Supplements*
- *New techniques and remedies*
- *Newsletters*

Your Wellness Partners,
Dr. Roni DeLuz and
James Hester

INDEX

2-day Weekend Cleanse, 2,
    156–57
  breaking the, 198
7-day Tune-Up, 2, 156–57
  breaking the, 197–98
21-day Diet Detox, 2–3, 81–100,
    156–57
  breaking the, 193–94
  the cleanup (stage one), 85–86
  connecting with higher self,
    94–96
  daily experience, 92–94
  daily schedule, 173, 175–81
  flushing out emotions, 90–91
  how it works, 82–85
  maintenance program, 194–97
  preparation for, 160
  repair and rebuild (stage two),
    86–89
  riding out healing crisis, 89–90
  testimonials, 97–100
  trouble-shooting tips, 181–84

abdominal bloating, 131
acid/fat connection, 64–67
acid reflux, 131
ADHD (attention deficit
    hyperactivity disorder), 25,
    202
aging, detoxing for, 3, 88
agricultural practices, 31–33
Agriculture, U.S. Department of
    (USDA), 83
allergies, 108, 122
aloe vera, 75, 122
American Biologics Clinic, 11–12
American Dietary Association,
    202

American eating habits, 30–41
  dead zone and, 34–36, 38
  gluttons for punishment, 38–41
American Gastrological
    Association (AGA), 130
American Institute of
    Hypnotherapy, 13
amylase, 35, 122
anaphylactic reactions, 175
antiaging, benefits of detoxing for,
    3, 88
antidepressants, 46, 183
antidiarrheals, 63–64
antioxidants, 87–89, 104–5
  berry drinks, 88–89, 120–21
Arnot's (Dr. Bob) Revolutionary
    diet, 71
arthritis, juice combination for,
    112
artificial sweeteners, 37–38, 202
Asian Spinach Soup, 205
aspartame, 37
athlete's foot, 48
Atkins diet, 71, 74–75
ATP (adenosine triphosphate), 119
attention deficit hyperactivity
    disorder (ADHD), 25, 202

Balch, Phyllis and James, 47
barley, 120
bathroom breaks, 62–63, 130–33
baths, detoxifying, 147
Beard, Hilary, 185–90
beets, 109
berry drinks, 88–89, 120–21
Black Cherry Kidney Flush, 146
blood pressure, high. See
    hypertension

blood sugar (glucose), 37–38,
    44–45, 47, 134
body
  ability to heal itself, 58–61
  pH of, 64–67
  ways we ignore our, 62–64
body mass index (BMI), 23
body/mind/spirit connection, 13,
    90–91
body odor, 42, 131
body temperature, extreme changes
    in, 182–83
body wraps, 149
bottled water, 84
bowel movements, 62–63, 130–33
Britto, Marvet, 17
broccoli, 31–32, 109
  Creamy Broccoli, 207
broccoli rabe, 109
Brown, Lorenzo and Jamie Foster,
    124
brown vegetables, 104
Buckley, Marcia, 78–80
Buckner, Eloise, 9, 11

cabbage, 109
cabinets, setting up your, 165–66
calcium, 202
calorie restriction, 56–57
calories, 23–24, 67–70
cancer, juice combination for, 112
Candida, 13, 48, 182
canned foods, 35–36, 159
canned juices, 102–3
carrots, 109
  Ginger Carrots, 207
  Sweet & Sour Carrot Dressing,
    210

cascara sagrada, 75
cauliflower, 110
cayenne pepper, 123
celery, 110
cells, 3, 58–61, 83
cellulase, 35, 122
cellulite treatments, 149–50
Center for Science in the Public Interest (CSPI), 39
central nervous system (CNS), 58–59
centrifugal juicers, 105, 106
CFS (chronic fatigue syndrome), 11, 14
chard, 110
chewing, 128, 193
Chi machine, 146–47
chlorophyll, 119
cholesterol, 44, 112
chronic fatigue syndrome (CFS), 11, 14
cigarette smoking, 47–48, 183
cilantro, 110
citrus juicers, 106
Clayton School of Natural Healing, 12–13
cleansing detoxification, 1–2, 76–77, 85–86. See also 2-day Weekend Cleanse; 7-day Tune-Up; 21-day Diet Detox
CNS (central nervous system), 58–59
coffee enemas, 145–46
colitis, 122
collard greens, 111
    Southern Collard Greens, 206
colon, 42, 128–29, 131–33
colon cleanses, 138–43
colon hydrotherapists, 139, 140
colonics (colon hydrotherapy), 9, 138–40
color of juices, 103–5
constipation, 42, 127, 129–30, 182
Consumer Reports, 33, 51
corn syrup, 36, 38
counter, setting up your, 165–66
cravings, 32–33, 175, 182
cucumbers, 110
    Cucumber Onion Dressing, 209
Curried Vegetables, 206

daily schedule, 173–81
    21-day Diet Detox, 173, 175–81
    planning your day, 167
    supplements, 174
    what to expect, 92–94
danger zone, avoiding the, 175
DDT, 76
dead zone, 34–36, 38
death ceremony, 8–9
DeLuz, Antonio (Tony), 11–12
DeLuz, Tony, Jr., 14
DeLuz, Toron, 14
department stores, 163
depression, 46, 183
detox (detoxing)
    benefits of, 3, 88
    dangers of, 77
    dieting vs., 74–76
    quiz, 6
detoxification programs, 1–2, 74–77. See also 2-day Weekend Cleanse; 7-day Tune-Up; 21-day Diet Detox
Detoxify or Die (Rogers), 27, 28, 29–30, 43
diabetes, 96
dieting
    culture of, 23–24, 67–70
    detoxing vs., 74–76
    pros and cons of popular diets, 71–74
    toxin's role in, 25
digestive aids, 42
digestive enzymes, 34–36, 102, 121–22
digestive system, 41–42, 128–33, 192–93
dioxins, 28
discount stores, 163
distilled water, 84
doctor, talking to your, 158
dopamine, 47–48
drinking water, 84, 137–38
    toxins in, 26–27, 28, 83
drinks
    berry, 88–89, 120–21
    green, 118–20
    protein, 123, 192
    shakes, recipes, 211–12
drugs, prescription, 46–47, 183
dry skin brushing, 147

eating habits, 30–41
    dead zone and, 34–36, 38
    gluttons for punishment, 38–41
Eat Right for Your Type diet, 72
E. coli, 34
elimination therapy, 127–51
    must-have treatments, 137–46
    nice treatments if you have time or money, 137, 149–51
    process of elimination, 128–36
    treatment schedule, 175–81
    want-to-have treatments, 137, 146–48
emotions, flushing out, 90–91
ending detox, 191–203
endocrine system, 59
enemas, 142–43
    coffee, 145–46
    colonics vs., 138–39
environmental hazards, 9–12, 83. See also toxins
environmental illness (EI), 12
Environmental Protection Agency (EPA), 28
Environmental Working Group (EWG), 28–29, 34
enzymes, 34–36, 102, 121–22
Equal, 37
essential fatty acids (EFAs), 201, 202
estrogen, 59
estrogen dominance, 46

family support, 158–59
fasting, 75–76
fat
    acid connection with, 64–67
    toxin's role in, 41–44
fatigue, 182
FDA (Food and Drug Administration), 26–27, 29, 40–41, 44, 121
feces, 132–33
fennel, 110
fevers, 63
fiber, 201–2
fibromyalgia, 11
Fit for Life Rotation diet, 72
flavored water, 164
flaxseed oils, 202
fluid retention, juice combination for, 112

fluoride poisoning, 26–27
food
    Americans' unhealthy
        relationship with, 30–41
    three levels of, 48–50
food allergies, 108, 122
Food and Drug Administration
        (FDA), 26–27, 29, 40–41, 44,
        121
food industry economics, 32–41
food labels, 33–34
Food Politics (Nestle), 40
Foods Standard Agency, 159
food-storage containers, 165
Forest, Rosalie, 124–26
free radicals, 87–88
free soup, 115, 165–66, 173
fresh foods, 35–36, 49, 56, 162
fresh juices. *See* juices
fruits, 88–89, 201
    berry drinks, 88–89, 120–21
    shopping list, 161
    washing, 34, 107–8

gallbladder, 134
gallbladder flush, 150–51
garlic, 46, 111
ginger, 111, 123
    Ginger Carrots, 207
glossary of terms, 213–16
glucose (blood sugar), 37–38,
        44–45, 47, 134
Glycemic Index diet, 72
goals, setting, 155–56
grazing, 54, 83
green drinks, 118–20
green peppers, 111
greens, 111
    Southern Collard Greens, 206
green teas, 165
green vegetables, 85, 104, 109–12,
        118–20
grocery shopping tips, 160–63, 203

HDL (high-density lipoprotein)
        cholesterol, 44, 112
headaches, 63
healing crisis, 19–20, 89–90
health-food stores, 163
heart disease, juice combination
        for, 112
herbal cleansing formula, 123

herbal teas, 162, 165
    colon cleansing, 141
    liver cleansing, 144
    parasite prevention, 183–84
Hester, Loretta, 97–98
high blood pressure. *See*
        hypertension
high-density nutritional
        supplements. *See* supplements
higher self, connecting with, 94–96
homeostasis, 61, 66
hormone imbalance, 45, 182–83
hormone replacement therapy
        (HRT), 46
hot flashes, 182–83
hunger pangs, 4, 175, 182
hydraulic presses, 107
hydrogenation, 43–44
hypertension, 96
    garlic capsules for, 46
    "white-coat," 55–56
hypnosis, 13
hypoglycemia, 134
hypothyroidism, 45

impotence, juice combination for,
        113
Indian tea, 165
ingredient labels, 33–34
inner wisdom, 56–61
insulin, 37–38, 44–45
Italian Green Beans, 208
Italian Naturally Dressing, 209
intestinal parasites. *See* parasites

Jenny Craig diet, 72–73
jock itch, 48
juicers, 105, 106–7
juices (juicing), 101–13
    characteristics of vegetables,
        108, 109–12
    for colon cleansing, 141
    by color, 103–5
    favorite combinations, 108,
        112–13
    for liver cleansing, 144
    maximizing vegetables' cleansing
        power, 102–3
    preparation, 105, 107–8

kale, 111
kidney cleanses, 146

kidneys, 8, 135
kitchen
    cleaning out your, 13—55, 159
    setting up for success, 64–66

laxatives, 127, 140–41
LDL (low-density lipoprotein)
        cholesterol, 44, 112
lead poisoning, 24–25, 28
lemon (lime) tea, 165
lipase, 35, 122
*Liquid Candy: How Soft Drinks Are
        Harming Americans' Health*
        (report), 39
liquid foods, 84, 86–87. *See also*
        drinks; juices; soups
liver, 134
liver cleanses (flushes), 123,
        144–46, 150–51
liver problems, juice for, 113
living foods, 35–36, 49, 56, 162
lodiquinol, 82
lymphatic system, 42, 135, 147–48
lymph drainage massage, 148

maintenance diet, 194–97,
        199–203
    eating more, 199
    shakes, 211–12
    shopping tips, 203
    what to add, 200–202
    what to avoid, 202
Martha's Vineyard Diet Detox. *See*
        21-day Diet Detox
Martha's Vineyard Holistic Retreat,
        14, 17–22
Martinez, Alberto, vii–ix, 81–82
massage, lymph drainage, 148
mass merchandisers, 163
Master Cleanse fast, 76
masticating juicers, 105, 106
meat marinades, 159
menopause, juice combination for,
        113
mercury poisoning, 25
metabolic resistance, 44–45
metabolism, 67–70
    sluggish, 47, 183
    toxin's role in, 25, 27
mind/body/spirit connection, 13,
        90–91
mustard greens, 111

must-have treatments, 137–46
    colonics, 138–40
    drinking water, 137–38
    enemas, 142–43, 145–46
    juice flush, 144
    kidney flush, 146
    laxatives, 140–41
    liver cleanses, 144–46
    treatment schedule, 175–81

National Association to Advance
    Fat Acceptance, 21
Natural Cures (Trudeau), 46–47
naturopathy, 12–13
Nestle, Marion, 39–41
nice treatments, 137, 149–51,
    175
nightshade vegetables, 108
Nutrasweet, 37
nutritional supplements. *See*
    supplements

oatmeal, 31–32
omega-3 fatty acids, 201, 202
omega-6 fatty acids, 201, 202
Omnivore's Dilemma, The (Pollan),
    32, 36, 38
onions, 111
    Cucumber Onion Dressing, 209
Orange-Cream Frappe, 211
orange vegetables, 104
organic foods, 48–51
    affordability of, 33, 51
Organic Trade Association, 48
overcivilized foods. *See* processed
    foods
overeating, 38–39, 64
oxygen, 57–58, 59
oxygen radical absorbance capacity
    (ORAC), 121

pancreas, 37–38, 44–45
pantry, setting up your, 165–66
parasites, 43, 81–82,
    tea for preventing, 183–84
parsnips, 111
PCBs (polychlorinated biphenyls),
    28
peaches, 121
peppers, green, 111
peristalsis, 132
Perricone diet, 73, 74–75

pH (potential hydrogenation),
    64–67
phagocytes, 129
photosynthesis, 57–58, 119
phthalates, 28
physician, talking to your, 158
phytonutrients, 104–5, 108–12,
    121
plastic bags, 165
Pollan, Michael, 32, 36, 38, 40
portion control, 30, 83
pregnant women, 96
prescription drugs, 46–47, 183
Prescription for Nutritional Healing
    (Balch), 47
Pritikin diet, 73, 74–75
probiotics, 140, 200–201
processed foods, 30–31, 34–36, 38,
    49, 66, 159
prostate problems, juice
    combination for, 113
protease, 35, 122
protein drinks, 123, 192
purple vegetables, 104

quiz, detox, 6

radishes, 112
Raw Foods diet, 73
Rebounders, 148
recipes, 205–12
    Asian Spinach Soup, 205
    Creamy Avocado Supreme, 211
    Creamy Broccoli, 207
    Cucumber Onion Dressing, 209
    Curried Vegetables, 206
    Ginger Carrots, 207
    Italian Green Beans, 208
    Italian Naturally Dressing, 209
    Orange-Cream Frappe, 211
    Southern Collard Greens, 206
    Spicy Green Bean Vinaigrette
        Dressing, 210
    Spicy Mustard Dressing, 210
    Sweet & Sour Carrot Dressing,
        210
    Yam Surprise, 212
recreational eating, 64
red vegetables, 104
refined foods. *See* processed foods
refrigerator, organization, 164
Regan, Judith, 15

Rogers, Sherry A., 27, 28, 29–30,
    43
roundworms, 45

saccharin, 37–38
safety concerns, 4
salad dressings, 159, 200
    recipes, 209–10
salad spinners, 164
salt, 95, 103, 202
saunas, 148
schedule. *See* daily schedule
senna tea, 75
setting goals, 155–56
shakes, recipes, 211–12
Shapiro's Picture Perfect diet,
    71–72
shopping tips, 160–63, 203
sick soil, 31–33
sick wheel, 8
Silverglade, Bruce, 41
skin, 135–36
skin rejuvenation, 3, 88
    dry skin brushing, 147
sleeping, 62
sluggish metabolism, 47, 183
small intestines, 128–29
smoking, 47–48, 183
sneezes (sneezing), 63
SOAP (subjective, objective,
    assessment, plan) notes, 11
sodium, 95, 103, 202
sodium laurel sulfate, in toothpaste,
    26
soft drinks, 39
soups, 113–15
    free, 115, 165–66, 173
    recipes, 205–8
South Beach Diet, 73–75
Southern Collard Greens, 206
soybeans, 31–32
spices, 161–62
Spicy Green Bean Vinaigrette
    Dressing, 210
Spicy Mustard Dressing, 210
spinach, 112
    Asian Spinach Soup, 205
spirulina, 120
Splenda, 38
spray-on tans, 26–27
stevia, 38
stomachaches, 42–43, 131

stool, 132–33
storing foods, 165
sucralose, 38
sugar substitutes, 37–38, 202
superfoods, 31–32, 121
supplements, 50, 85–86, 117–26.
     See also drinks
   aloe vera, 75, 122
   daily schedule, 174
   digestive enzymes, 121–22
   herbal cleansing formula, 123
   storing near you, 166–67
support system, 158–59
sweeteners, artificial, 37–38, 202
Sweet & Sour Carrot Dressing, 210
Sweet'N Low, 37–38
sweet potatoes, 112
syndrome X, 44–45

teas, 162, 165
   colon cleansing, 141
   liver cleansing, 144
   parasite prevention, 183–84
tea-tree oil, 85
testosterone, 59
Thompson, Judi, 168–71
thrush, 48
thyroxin, 45
tomatoes, 112
toothpaste, 26
toxic overload, 28–29, 43
toxins, 24–30
   quiz, 6
   role in weight gain, 41–44

trans fats, 43–44
Trezanowski, Geri, 98–99
triturating juicers, 106
Trudeau, Kevin, 46–47
Tupperware, 165
turnip greens, 111
turnips, 112

ulcers, juice combination for, 113
undereating, 56–57
upset stomach, 42–43, 131
urinary incontinence, 62–63
USDA (U.S. Department of
     Agriculture), 83

vaginal yeast infections, 48
vegetables. *See also* juices; recipes;
     soups; *and specific vegetables*
   characteristics of, 108, 109–12
   cleaning, 34, 107–8, 164
   color of, 103–5
   shopping list, 161
vitamin C, 121

Walsh, Joan, 99–100
want-to-have treatments, 137,
     146–48
   Chi machine, 146–47
   detoxifying bath, 147
   dry skin brushing, 147
   lymph drainage massage, 147–48
   Rebounder, 148
   sauna, 148
   treatment schedule, 175–81

washing produce, 34, 107–8, 164
water, 84, 137–38
   toxins in, 26–27, 28, 83
weekend detox. *See* 2-day Weekend
     Cleanse
week-long detox. *See* 7-day Tune-
     Up
weight gain
   prescription drug's role in, 46–47
   toxin's role in, 25
weight-loss programs. *See* 2-day
     Weekend Cleanse; 7-day
     Tune-Up; 21-day Diet Detox
weight maintenance, 194–97,
     199–203
   shakes, 211–12
   shopping tips, 203
   what to add, 200–202
   what to avoid, 202
Weight Watchers diet, 74
wheatgrass, 107, 118–19, 144
"white-coat" hypertension, 55–56
white vegetables, 104
Whole Foods, 48, 50
Williams, Deborah, 9, 17
Windemere Nursing and
     Rehabilitation Center, 14
work days, 167

Yam Surprise, 212
yeast overgrowth, 48
yellow vegetables, 104

Zone diet, 74